Praise for *More Scripts and Strategies in Hypnotherapy*

Even when I use regression or parts therapy, suggestions and imagery are used at both the first and last session ... so there is always a place for well written scripts. Lynda Hudson's *More Scripts and Strategies in Hypnotherapy* is filled with useful ideas. Her hypnotic phrases included in the opening chapter are so excellent that they would likely be praised by Erickson himself! She blends many other metaphors throughout her book. Many of Hudson's offerings are slanted for medical uses of hypnosis, which is great for hypnotherapists who work with medical referrals. The author's 'soothing liquid calm' for IBS is masterful; and she also offers some unique scripts for pain management, as well as for pregnancy and childbirth.
Roy Hunter, published author of several hypnosis texts

Lynda Hudson's latest book, *More Scripts and Strategies*, is deliciously broad in scope, covering a wide range of topics. It is a phenomenal teaching tool with in-depth information and explanations and is written with great clarity. As a hypnotherapy instructor, I especially appreciate the suggestion boxes of variations, adaptations and recommendations. They provide additional teaching for both the novice and the established hypnotherapist. A highly recommended, well-written book of scripts!
Katherine Zimmerman, author, *Hypnotherapy Scripts, Vol. II*

Perhaps best known for her work with children, Lynda Hudson now uses her extensive therapeutic knowledge and scripting skills to encompass adults, producing a unique and innovative book that steps beyond the bounds of the usual collection of scripts. Far from repeating what is already on the shelves, she has looked for what is missing and has admirably filled the gaps. With each script being analysed in detail we are left in no doubt as to the therapeutic meaning and implication of every individual component. These factors and more combine to make *More Scripts and Strategies in Hypnotherapy* stand out as an original and exciting inclusion in the pantheon of script books, one that has plenty to impart to even the most experienced of therapists.
Peter Mabbutt FBSCH, FBAMH, CEO/Director of Studies, London College of Clinical Hypnosis

This excellent book by Lynda Hudson somehow manages to weave influences from all kinds of diverse sources into an exciting coherent whole. It is everything you would want of a new hypnotherapy sourcebook for students and practitioners – fresh, practical and accessible. An important contribution to the development of hypnotherapy scripting, *More Scripts & Strategies in Hypnotherapy* synthesises the best of traditional approaches with important new developments emerging across a range of different areas.

Combining practical accessibility with theoretical sophistication, this book will be invaluable reading for beginning therapists and experienced clinicians. The individual scripts presented and the self-practice/self-reflection trajectories will no doubt support continuous professional development in this area.

The author provides a clear rationale for the inclusion of key scripted words and phrases and discusses the importance of the therapist taking into account their own beliefs and emotions in formulating each case.

Andy Young RMN, LLB(Hons), LLM, PG Cert Hed, Senior Lecturer in Mental Health Nursing, Sheffield Hallam University

I was delighted when, in 2009 came the book *Scripts and Strategies in Hypnotherapy with Children*. This book was expertly written by Lynda Hudson. I remember well reviewing this book which was certainly an excellent addition to any practitioner's book shelf. Most certainly it is a book which is proving, rightfully so, to be a bestseller.

Now Crown House have done it again! I am delighted that we now have *More Scripts and Strategies in Hypnotherapy* penned, once again, expertly and compassionately by Lynda Hudson. The book, as its name suggests, follows on in the footsteps of Roger Allen, but has its own personal stamp and form.

The book demonstrates fully the author's deep understanding of the subject and also of the needs of both the therapist and the clients. It has been well researched and thoughtfully compiled and contains a wealth of invaluable advice, guidance and information for the therapist as s/he sets out upon the healing mission, however experienced they may be.

The style is clear and uncluttered and, where appropriate, explanation is given to make sure that the reader is able to gain full benefit from the material. This presentation is geared for practical work. It is thought provoking. This is material you will look at again and again as you build up your own personal resources. Like an excellent novel too it is one of those books you just can't put down. If you want a ready made script for a particular problem it is there and can be used as it is. However I feel that the work stimulates the practitioner to think and amend and make the material more suited to his or her own personal style of delivery.

Having had a pre-production copy of this I have been able to use some of the material with my own patients. It was very well received and very easy to work with and build on. Material this time has been composed to cover anxiety, panic, phobias and moderate depression. I have used the section on sleep and this was most effective.

Lynda talks about various sexual issues with great care and compassion and the book can be used by the therapist with confidence in an area from which many people shy away.
The IBS section is especially worthy of note and I have found that this is well received by patients. Now I am pleased to have a wider selection of material to develop my own work from. There is work on childbirth, surgery and pain, as well as enhancing performance in sport and business. It really is a cornucopia of sheer excellence.

I assure you, here is a book that the whole of our profession has been waiting for. I feel that we cannot afford to be without it as it inspires confidence and delivers the best of material and is written by someone who really understands us, the therapists, what we need and how we tick, as well as having the deepest interests of the clients at heart.
David Slater BA, DHyp, MHA(RegHyp), MASC, DCS, MGSCT, Clinical Hypnotherapist and Counsellor

As I read Hudson's work I noticed that she covers both script and hypnotherapy strategy elements on each page. Each page is vertically split so that one part of the page is the prescribed script and the other part of the page contains Hudson's guidance regarding the professional hypnotherapy strategy in use. This ingenious presentation is a wonderful technique. It keeps you very aware of the strategies which are annotated alongside the actual script. The core hypnotic strategies can help you to develop your own style and the scripts are designed to build your repertoire of hypnotic language, strategies and attitude.

I also noticed I could apply each of the various scripts to a number of situations I was dealing with in my varied practice. I am excited and so happy that this book is here.
Deborah Rose, Hypnotherapist for www.StressFreecaringintheCity

More Scripts and Strategies is a treasure trove for any hypnotherapist looking for new inspiration and ideas. Covering a wide range of issues from basic relaxation to childbirth, sports and surgery, it is fully comprehensive in the subjects covered, yet wonderfully concise in delivery. Each script is accompanied by easy to follow instructions for timing and delivery, along with many other helpful suggestions throughout. As Lynda points out in her preface different clients need different strategies – it simply isn't 'one size fits all'; with that in mind this book is an absolute must.
Daragh O'Sullivan ICHP PGA

Until now Roger Allen's book (The Complete Works) has provided more script and idea sources for my hypnotherapy practice than any other reference material. It was indeed a very pleasant surprise to read Lynda Hudson's *More Scripts and Strategies in Hypnotherapy*. This is a veritable hypnotherapy encyclopaedia with scripts and succinct notes for a very wide range of problems. I recommend it as an essential reference book.
Barry Shirley DCH, Dip Couns, DRM, MASCH, MAHA, MACA, MATMS

The clarity, creativity and practicality of Lynda's *Scripts and Strategies* ensure it's a must for all hypnotherapists, both experienced and novice. Her expertise and exceptional imaginative flair are displayed throughout the scripts. Succinct explanations and therapy options add insight and direction for the practitioner.
   I would highly recommend this book.
Bernadette Rizzo, Vice President of the Australian Hypnotherapists Association

More Scripts and Strategies in Hypnotherapy

Lynda Hudson

Crown House Publishing Limited
www.crownhouse.co.uk
www.crownhousepublishing.com

First published by

Crown House Publishing Ltd
Crown Buildings, Bancyfelin, Carmarthen, Wales, SA33 5ND, UK
www.crownhouse.co.uk

and

Crown House Publishing Company LLC
6 Trowbridge Drive, Suite 5, Bethel, CT 06801-2858, USA
www.crownhousepublishing.com

First published 2010. Reprinted 2012.

British Library Cataloguing-in-Publication Data
A catalogue entry for this book is available
from the British Library.

13 Digit ISBN 978-184590391-6

LCCN 2009936671

Printed and bound in the UK by
Bell & Bain Ltd, Glasgow

For
Jonathon,
Tim and Frances

Table of Contents

i

Acknowledgements

In writing this book I have had enormous support from my dear husband, John(athon), and my good friend and colleague Anne Lesley Marshall. I would like both of them to know how much I appreciate their wonderful support throughout, both practical and emotional.

Jonathon:

Thank you for your patient reading and rereading every word of these scripts, not once but several times over.

Thank you also for your invaluable comments, advice, ideas and your meticulous proofreading.

Thank you for your belief in me.

(Thank you for your nurturing and ensuring that we didn't go hungry while I wrote!)

Anne:

Thank you for reading and commenting on these scripts and offering your very helpful opinions and suggestions.

I particularly appreciate your very generous advice and suggestions in regard to the section on childbirth. Your midwifery experience has been invaluable to me.

As you have been writing your own book on coaching people to better health, I know how precious your time has been and you have given it to me most generously.

I am also indebted to Dr Anna Zohrabian, Medical Principal of the London College of Clinical Hypnosis, for checking my sections of medical notes and offering extra suggestions. Thank you, Anna.

A big thank you goes to Angela Everitt for trialling many of my scripts and for her helpful comments. Thanks also to John Hempstead, Christa McKinnon and all other colleagues and peers who gave me their comments.

Thanks also go to the team at Crown House; to David, once again for trusting me and giving me no constraints in writing this book, to Beverley and Rosalie for their helpful editing and marketing on my behalf, always so patient and good humoured, and also to Peter for copy-editing and Tom for the cover design.

Introduction

First and foremost I would like to say what an enormous privilege it is to be asked to write this latest volume in the Scripts and Strategies series. I am well aware of the responsibility I have taken on in following in the footsteps of Roger Allen, whose previous volumes have been such an invaluable resource for hypnotherapists all over the world. Naturally our styles will differ, but I hope this volume will complement Roger's first two volumes.

More Scripts and Strategies in Hypnotherapy is a compendium of scripts intended to complement Roger Allen's original *Scripts and Strategies in Hypnotherapy*. This means that some traditional areas such as smoking or weight do not appear in this volume since they were very well covered in Roger's book and also in many other books. I have, however, included certain conditions or problems which have been covered previously, in particular anxiety, because unfortunately I see more and more patients these days for conditions which are stress and anxiety based and I believe there is a continuing demand from therapists for different scripts designed to relieve these symptoms.

As hypnotherapy becomes better known and understood by the general public it seems that there is more of a demand for help with issues that fall outside the more well known categories of giving up smoking, weight management and relief from anxiety. Consequently I have tried to fulfil a requirement for scripts which deal with issues such as vocal and motor tics, essential tremor, sexual issues, antenatal, childbirth and post-natal concerns to name but a few. There is a substantial section which deals with coping with pain, taking into account emotional and psychological elements as well as physical aspects. There are also several scripts which deal with the different aspects of irritable bowel syndrome (IBS) which is a condition which has been shown to have a very good response to hypnotherapy. Indeed, in some hospitals nowadays hypnotherapy has become the treatment of choice for IBS.

Very broadly the issues fall into categories of Mental, Emotional and Physical Health and Well-being, Enhanced Business Performance,

Sports and Arts Performance and Public Speaking. The latter includes presentation giving and attending interviews which are well recognized sources of enormous stress to many people in all walks of life. Nevertheless there are many topics which do not fall neatly into the above categories so I decided not to try to 'force' them unnaturally into specific section headings. I believe that you, the therapist, will scan the table of contents for the particular issue you wish to address. If you do not immediately find the condition you are seeking, it could be worthwhile your checking the small sections which appear in most chapters suggesting variations, adaptations and recommendations since many of the scripts can be adapted to other issues.

The scripts vary considerably in topic and metaphor so as to appeal to a wide range of age groups, interests, personalities and preferred approaches of both client and clinician. There are healing lakes, cleansing fountains, stepping stones across a stream to a better future and there are mental computers for programming mind and body, mental biofeedback machines and problem-fixing applications to download from the internet. There are healing dreams, inner conversations and parcels to be unwrapped to release unwanted layers of pain. There are also very straightforward, down-to-earth direct suggestions and visualizations of successful outcomes.

I have adopted a format which is a little different from both Roger's original *Scripts and Strategies in Hypnotherapy* and my own *Scripts and Strategies in Hypnotherapy for Children*. The new format allows comments to the therapist alongside the script to give some insight into my thinking; in some cases the comment draws attention to hypnotic devices or explains specific wording, and in other cases it suggests emphasis in the use of the voice or a way to adapt the script to suit the individual client. Thus, although this is fundamentally a compendium of scripts intended for trained hypnotherapists, I have tried to offer the reader something a little over and above a bare script. For the newer therapist it can also act as a teaching tool, pointing out useful presuppositions, embedded commands, generalizations, truisms and language chosen to invoke different sensory experience which otherwise might not be recognized. For the more experienced clinician it offers reminders, explanations and choices. For the hypnotherapy instructor it gives useful examples of theory put into practice and for clinical supervision it provides a basis for reflection and discussion. I would emphasize once again however that the collection first and foremost is intended as a practical sourcebook for practising clinicians whether recently trained or very experienced.

The scripts vary in length and style in order to suit different problems, situations and personalities and stem from years of experience in private practice. Colleagues have also been generous in reading, commenting and, in some cases, trialling scripts more or less as they stand, and, in others, adapting them to suit their own style and that of the individual client. My overriding message to you is to adapt any script to your own way of working. Please feel free to lengthen, shorten and extemporize as you see fit. Personally I am a great believer in embedded commands/suggestions and you will find many of these throughout the scripts, mostly in italics, so be aware of these when you adapt and reword.

There are several instances where the client is asked to carry out a mental activity or is asked to agree to a proposition which will move them in their desired direction. They are given pause for thought and normally my presupposition is that the suggestion will be accepted. In a collection of general scripts it is impossible to account for every response a client might have but it should be born in mind that it may be necessary to reframe ideas and suggestions, include some parts negotiation, or reconsider goals. In this case of course there will be a need to adapt the script and extemporise as appropriate. I have included suggestions for variations, adaptations and recommendations where I feel they may be helpful.

Generally, with certain exceptions, I have not included inductions in the main body of the script, although sometimes I have suggested that one particular style would be more appropriate than another. In some cases just a conversational lead into the script would be fine, and in others, something deeper or more dramatically convincing would be helpful. In a couple of cases where inductions appear as part of the script, they have also been included in the *Inductions* section itself. This section is fairly brief as many inductions were given in Roger's collection and they abound elsewhere. 'Light' inductions may often, but not always, be more suited to the workplace or sports coaching environment. Incidentally, the ideas in both these sections can easily be adapted and used in a personal setting too; procrastination, for example, is certainly not exclusive to the world of business.

I have offered a greater selection of reorientations since I think this is an area not so well represented in other collections and I believe it is an important opportunity to add suggestions for well-being, ongoing change and progress at the unconscious level. There are reorientations with renewal of hope particularly suitable for patients suffering from pain or illness, others which are especially energizing and others that encourage the listener to put plans to into action. Suggestions for reintegration of parts, mild confusion, partial amnesia or removal of trance phenomena are included in different endings. Some of these suggestions of course are optional but sometimes they will be essential before returning to full conscious awareness of the present moment.

My assumption is that normally problems will require more than one treatment session, so one script is not intended to deal with a problem outright, particularly if it is complex or long-standing. Some scripts will be more appropriate for initial sessions whereas others will provide solid reinforcement.

There are certain issues, however, such as examination nerves, where I have personally found one session to be easily enough. By the way, since in my former career I was a language teacher, director of studies and teacher trainer, I felt compelled to add a couple of suggestions for examination technique in addition to dealing with the performance anxiety aspect. It also means that I am aware of the sheer terror experienced by some teachers when having to undergo inspections or lesson observation/assessments; hence a script to deal with that issue!

Talking of education, here in the UK at least, teaching approaches have come, gone and come back again in popularity over the years, with proponents of one method claiming it is the best or the only one to get results. I have a feeling that it is somewhat similar in the field of therapy but it is my belief that different clinicians help their patients achieve remarkable results through completely different approaches if they have a genuine and passionate belief in them. The approach, needless to say, has to be right for the patient and therapist alike. I know it should go without saying, but forgive me if I say it anyway, that good listening and rapport are crucial.

So, of course, are trust and respect, and wholehearted, mutual belief in the method, together with the skill and compassion of the therapist. To that end, this collection contains scripts which involve both direct and indirect suggestion, metaphor, complexity and simplicity, dissociation from a feeling and association into a feeling - although I would add, not all at the same time!

Earlier I said that I have tried to offer something a little over and above the actual script itself. In addition to the accompanying comments, I have also provided at the outset a chapter setting out some useful hypnotic language and expressions to help with devising your own scripts or adapting those contained in this volume. They contain examples, which can be mixed and matched, of presuppositions of success and positive intent, generalizations, suggestions phrased as questions, phrases covering all possibilities of response and various other expressions which lead to the acceptance of a therapeutic idea.

There are also several short sections which provide brief information or points to bear in mind when selecting or adapting a script, or even choosing whether to treat at all before medical diagnosis and referral. For some of you this will just serve as a reminder and for others it may be a pointer to research a condition further before treatment. Where it refers to medical or psychological topics, please be aware that the information is not intended to cover the topic in depth, nor be sufficient on its own, nor to replace medical advice.

Conventions and expressions

I use the words *patient* and *client* more or less interchangeably to reflect the different settings where you may practise, for example, hospital or private therapy.

I use the term 'unconscious mind' to refer to the processes which are happening outside of our conscious awareness. Memories and emotions can drive or influence our behaviour even when we are not consciously aware of them, or, in some cases, cannot consciously face them. There have been many theories concerning the unconscious mind, those of Freud, Lacan and Jung to name but a few, and of course there are some theorists who believe that the existence of an unconscious mind is simply a myth. In hypnotherapy the unconscious is certainly a useful concept that we can make use of whether through regressions, parts work, or suggestion in order to help a client become more aware of underlying causes of unwanted behaviour and then deal with them more effectively. Some people may prefer to use the term 'subconscious', particularly to refer to thoughts or feelings very easily brought into conscious awareness, while others may find that the term 'inner mind' is preferable. Please adapt, or even omit, specific terminology in order to fit with your own beliefs and, perhaps more importantly, those of your client.

I use the terms 'associated' and 'dissociated' in the NLP tradition. The former, having a sense of being inside an experience, seeing it thorough one's own eyes and fully experiencing it, and the latter experiencing it from a more detached point of view as if seeing or thinking of oneself in a situation at one step removed from it.

I have generally used the words *future pace* to mean *mental rehearsal* or *pseudo-orientation in time*.

Comments to the therapist are normally added on the right-hand side of the page and are in bold. Occasionally, for convenience, they also occur in the main body of the script.

Pauses in the script are indicated by the ellipsis symbol ... and a longer pause by [Pause].

Italics are used to show where to use additional emphasis in your voice in order to highlight embedded commands or particularly important phrases.

In some generic scripts examples have been underscored to indicate that they need to be replaced when dealing with other presenting problems.

Parenthesized phrases may indicate either that they need to be spoken rather like an aside (so to speak) or as an option that should be omitted if not relevant. I hope this will be obvious from the text itself.

To my non-British readers

As I am English and live in London, I have largely used British English vocabulary, spelling and expressions, for example in both the areas of work and childbirth here in the UK we have *labour* whereas in the USA and other countries you have *labor*. We use *practice* for the noun and *practise* for the verb. We have *got* and you have *gotten* and so it goes on. So please, be patient and just mentally adapt spellings and change expressions as you go along. Thank you for your understanding.

Lynda Hudson
March 2010

Hypnotic Language

Useful phrases and presuppositions

I wonder whether/if	it will surprise you …
Quite probably/possibly	you'll be curious …
In all probability	you'll enjoy …
Perhaps/maybe	you've noticed before
It might be that	you'll drift and dream or focus on every word
	you'll be reminded of a time when …
	you'll be pleased/amazed/surprised/fascinated/interested to notice …
	you'll be surprised to discover that …
I wonder how quickly/soon/easily	you'll find yourself becoming …
	you'll notice yourself enjoying …
I invite you to	take a little time to explore
I'd like you to	discover something interesting/meaningful
I want you to	
I'd like to suggest that you	have a new/interesting/experience
And why not allow yourself to	
Can you/you can notice	how these changes in you will affect your family/friends
Can you/you can be pleased	
	that not only you but all those people around you are benefitting from your new behaviour
And maybe/perhaps you'll enjoy	noticing/discovering/finding/experiencing/drifting deeper/daydreaming/relaxing in a new way
It's nice/comforting/interesting/fascinating/encouraging/amusing/surprising to	discover/know/find/notice …
	become aware of inner thoughts and dreams

Some people	relax immediately
And people can	become very deeply relaxed
And it's just fine/all right/okay to	get a sense of
	find this is a very powerful/deeply moving/insightful experience
	experience this in whatever way is right for you
	stay very lightly relaxed as you make some profound changes
All that really matters right now is for you to	learn/experience this/enjoy this fully
All that's really important is to	keep all these insights in a place in you where your unconscious will make use of them in the best possible way for you
All that need concern you is to	
And your unconscious mind can enable you to	
Give yourself the opportunity to	
What's important/interesting now is the ability of your mind to	
And, if you wish, you can	
You'll be drawn to	
You don't need to be concerned if	this doesn't *happen immediately/ straightaway* for it will *happen at the right time for you*

And would you be willing to experience	a sense of increasing pleasure/relaxation/awareness
It may be that you're already aware of	an internal/unconscious desire to change
The really important thing is to be fully aware of	sensations of calm and comfort spreading around your body
And you can let yourself become more and more aware of	inner thoughts and feelings long, long forgotten
And you can begin by allowing/noticing	intriguing ideas that you can make use of
Perhaps noticing	a thought that can change everything
Perhaps beginning to notice	ideas beginning to develop
Maybe it will surprise you to notice	
Notice yourself noticing	
Perhaps you wouldn't mind noticing	
Are you noticing *yet*	
Becoming gradually, or perhaps suddenly, aware of	
And this can happen here	sooner than you expected/more easily than you thought it could, couldn't it?
And this may happen	now, or later as you sleep, or in the morning as you wake, and in the days and weeks that follow
And you can do/experience this	in a way that meets your needs at this time/in your own special way
It's going to be a delight to achieve this	not in my way, not in anyone else's way ... but in your own way
Now, of course, I don't know, and I don't need to know, exactly	when you first were aware of this response/feeling
You yourself may not yet know	which of your internal resources are best to use right now/in this case
And you begin to wonder	which of your qualities/inner resources will be most useful to you now
	when/how you will first notice how much stronger you feel

Perhaps even taking certain pride/delight in And you will be surprised, perhaps, at		your ability/willingness/determination/decision to …
And will you surprise yourself by enjoying yourself or enjoy yourself by surprising yourself		as all these changes occur?
You already know how to … You have always known that you could …		but I wonder if you have been able to really appreciate this ability as you can right now
One of the things I'd like you to discover is One of the first things you can become aware of is And I think you're going to enjoy being surprised by You'll be fascinated by And as that occurs, you really can't help but notice		a sense of wonderment/ease/contentment/eagerness/excitement/satisfaction how much you really want to make those changes now
The harder you try to stay awake		the more sleep will overtake you
The more you try to resist the sensations of trance/of sexual desire/arousal		the more the feelings will develop
It's not necessary to You don't need to It's not important to You may not expect to	right now just at the moment	*make all the changes … just to give them your full consideration* *go into a really deep level of trance*
And you don't even have to know consciously	how your mind is becoming more receptive … how your mind will experience [x] or [y] … how to do this …	it can all happen at the unconscious level you can trust your unconscious mind to do it all for you you can just get a sense of it beginning within
So that it's almost as if I don't know if you're aware of these changes yet, and in one way it doesn't really matter, for		what is really important is that the changes have taken place deep within you

And it appears that	things have been changing already
And, in an interesting way, you'll discover that	you have been noticing
Even perhaps amusing yourself as you discover	some of these things have already been happening
And it's very rewarding to know that	these changes are occurring because of your own efforts/insights
And, you, of course, know better than anyone else that	
And that will probably remind you of	other experiences, and other feelings you've had that are empowering
And letting yourself begin to notice *one* thing ... or maybe more than one thing	that's *about to happen*
	that's already changed
Is this the *first time* you've noticed, or have you noticed before, that	you are seeing things more clearly?
	you are being more objective?
	you are feeling more positive/optimistic?
	you are behaving more confidently?
And this may happen	very soon, in fact it may have already happened at the unconscious level and is just waiting for your conscious mind to become aware of it
	over the next few days and weeks, or overnight or right now or later today ... the important thing is that it will happen at the perfect time for you
And *because* you are able to relax a little more deeply now	your unconscious mind will automatically take on the suggestions
And *because* you have relaxed more deeply and become more and more receptive	
And because you have decided to let go of that old way of thinking	
And *if* you allow yourself to relax just a little more	*then* you will/may begin to notice ...
As you allow yourself to focus completely on the sound of my voice	*then* you will find yourself in a place of even greater relaxation
And that feeling of inner calm/sense of inner focus/sense of achievement/deeper relaxation/letting go	*makes you* aware that you have genuinely made some changes
	makes you consider the opportunities that have opened up to you

Anxiety, Panic, Phobias

Ratio breathing

This can be used as an induction or a deepener, or simply a short therapeutic activity in its own right.

It is useful to teach the technique before you begin the script and explain how it gives the client control over their breathing.

Settle yourself comfortably in the chair and let your eyes close and begin to imagine that the air around you is a wonderful colour of calm and comfort ... I wonder what colour that would be ... and as I count from 1 to 3 ... I'd like you to breathe in through your nose that wonderful calming, comforting colour so it spreads throughout your whole body ... are you ready? ... In 2, 3 ... Out 2, 3, 4, 5, 6 ... In 2, 3 ... Out 2, 3, 4, 5, 6 ... and *each time you breathe out through your nose, you can breathe out any tension in your body* ... you can even look inside and notice the colour of that tension and ... as we count out ... just breathe out that colour ... Out 2, 3, 4, 5, 6 ... *breathe away any tension in your mind* ... that's right .... breathing. In 2, 3 ... Out 2, 3, 4, 5, 6 ... In 2, 3 ... Out 2, 3, 4, 5, 6 ... and *each time you do this ... your level of calm and comfort increases* ... you *become more and more relaxed ... you become more and more in control of your relaxation* ... and this *will continue as we go on.*

This script makes use of, the simple controlled breathing technique where you breathe in to the count of 3 and out to the count of 6, or in to the count of 4 and out to the count of 8

The addition of the colour to the breathing adds to feelings of calm and takes the focus off the body

Each time you begin counting again, match the count to their breathing

Using the words 'more in control of your relaxation' gives the patient a sense of being in control

So ... as you've been breathing in the calm to the count of three and breathing out the tension to the count of six ... have you been noticing just *how very calming this is*? ... How it *gives you control over your breathing and control over your feelings* ... and every time you do this ... always remembering to *breathe only through your nose* ... you will strengthen your ability to *stay calm and in control in any situation* ... you have a tool you can use anywhere ... any time ... you want to *increase your calm and increase your control.* So in a moment or two I'm going to begin

This can be taught in or out of trance as a coping mechanism to control anxious feelings

Breathing through the nose gives additional control and helps to avoid hyperventilation

6

the counting again and then I'm going to allow you to continue your own inner counting … keeping the rhythm … breathing in through your nose and out through your nose … breathing in the calm … and breathing out the tension … as I stay silent for a while … that's it … ready … In 2, 3 … Out 2, 3, 4, 5, 6 … In 2, 3 … Out 2, 3, 4, 5, 6 … breathing in the colour of calm … breathing out the colour of tension … In 2, 3 … Out 2, 3, 4, 5, 6 … breathe away any tension in your mind … that's right.

Inner counting also provides a form of distraction from focus on the body or focus on fear

Stay silent for about a minute as you allow the client to continue the rhythm and after a while restart the counting in time with their breathing

Excellent job … I want you to know that the more you practise this at home … the more you strengthen the power of this ratio breathing which gives you calm and control in any situation … any time … any place … with anybody you're with … or just calmly on your own … calm and control. That's right.

It is useful to set this as a homework activity to practise on a daily basis to reinforce using ratio breathing as a calming coping mechanism

Go to further therapeutic suggestions, or ego strengthening and trance reorientation as appropriate

Variations, Adaptations and Recommendations

Ratio Breathing is best carried out while breathing through the nose, as this will slow down and regulate the breathing. It is a useful technique to teach patients to use if they have a tendency to panic. A frequent response to anxiety is for people to feel that they can't get enough air and then they open their mouths to catch their breath and begin to hyperventilate (over-breathe). This hyperventilation in itself can cause major panicky feelings in their body and in their minds too. Ratio breathing can help restore the delicate balance of oxygen and CO_2 in the blood necessary for normal functioning.

Using the above as an induction has a twofold effect: it is calming and relaxing in itself and, at the same time, the patient is being taught an invaluable technique to use on their own. It is probably best only to tell them afterwards that it can be a coping technique for panic in order to avoid their becoming anxious about needing to learn it in the first place!

Rewind procedure

There are many variations on this theme which is based on dissociation and guided visualisation in a way which breaks up the original coding of the memory in the brain. We remember things in words, sounds, pictures, feelings, and sometimes smells and tastes too, and we normally remember them in the sequence they occurred. If we play about with the sequencing, the colours, the size, and any other variable that you can think of, the memory trace stored in our brains and any associated negative feelings are altered, in some cases quite dramatically. This is a useful first intervention for situations where there have been one or more specific frightening events which have triggered anxiety, panic or phobias. The Rewind Procedure can be carried out with or without formal trance.

When you choose to use this type of intervention with a tragic incident, it would clearly be inappropriate to use some of the suggestions for humorous modality change such as using cartoons.

Demonstrate the procedure of 'rewinding imagery' with a memory which has no upsetting content and will be clear in client's minds, such as their journey to see you.

Summary of Rewind Procedure

1. Prepare to turn the frightening event into a film/movie/ sequence on a computer screen and establish a safe beginning and a safe end.

2. See the sequence through on the screen from beginning to end (Optional: create further dissociation by sitting above/beside self to watch whole process). Freeze-frame the safe end scene.

3. Run the sequence backwards as if on rewind mode, emphasizing the safe end and safe beginning. Blank out the screen.

4. Repeat Rewind Procedure, changing modalities of speed, size, colour, cartoons etc., blanking out the screen between each rewind.

5. Optional: step into the end scene of the sequence (associated) and rewind it again.

6. Run it forwards again from the beginning, ensuring that the client behaves as they would prefer to have done (dissociated). Repeat this action until no further improvements can be made and the client reports that previous negative feelings have been eliminated or significantly reduced.

7. Step into the picture and go through the event from beginning to end, noticing the feelings of confidence and calm (associated).

Generic rewind template

Eliminate or lessen the effect of a previously experienced frightening event, phobic response or panic attack

This script may be used with phobic responses, panic attack and milder anxiety too. It can also be adapted for use with a traumatic or tragic situation where you would employ more dissociative techniques and avoid insensitive humour. It makes use of 'one-stage dissociation' by asking the client to see, as a mental movie/ film, a previously experienced frightening event which had either caused or reinforced an anxiety, phobic response or panic attack. It then employs 'two-stage dissociation' by having the client's observant part float out of the body and view the event from a doubly-dissociated perspective. It can be used either within a formal deep trance framework or as an informal and conversational light trance framework, getting feedback as you go along.

It is important to establish the safe start and end scenes of the mental movie before you start the script so the client has very clear, safe and calm anchor points.

Before embarking on the use of the script, you might like to experiment, merely conversationally, with your patient, with changing modalities of a different memory to see whether changing the size, colour, etc, of an internal image has positive or negative effects.

I'd like you to be aware of yourself sitting comfortably here in the chair just about to switch on your imaginary remote control to view your imaginary television/computer screen … and then do a rather unusual thing … let the part of you *that is very good at observing* float up and sit down beside you and observe you watching the movie which is about to begin.	**Watching a screen provides one-stage dissociation. Floating out a part from the body lends further distance from the event**
	Presupposition that 'there is a part of you that is very good at observing'
Tell me when you're there … good.	**Compliance with the request demonstrates participation in the process**
So, just as we discussed earlier … the opening scene of your movie is the one before you <u>got on the train/bus</u> where *you are feeling absolutely safe and*	**You will have elicited safe starting and end points**

10

fine/calm/normal. Got that image? Good … now run that movie through from beginning to end and tell me when you've got/gotten to the end scene where *you are, once more, feeling perfectly safe* and <u>back in the house/on the platform/waiting at the bus station</u> … just wherever *you are feeling perfectly safe and secure* … good … very well done indeed/good job. Now fill that screen with an incredibly bright light for a moment so you *see only light* and nothing else before we begin to *change all those old unwanted feelings into more positive ones* … great

Filling the screen with light helps the client to break any emotional state and not carry over any possible negative feelings into the next activity

Now get that very safe final scene up on the screen once again and then press the rewind switch on the (imaginary) remote control in your hand and *watch it all speeding backwards* from the end to the beginning … and notice how it's at triple speed and everything is happening in that rather funny jerky way that *lends a whole new perspective on everything/that lets you see things in a completely different way … and gives you a totally different feeling about it* … let me know when you are back at the opening scene of the movie where you *feel perfectly safe and at ease*. Well done. Now here's the remarkable thing … when you do that, you *break up* not only *the sequence of events* in your mind but you *break up the feelings* of that old memory that you *used* to carry around so that you *change the effect completely* … so you *get a totally different and reasonable response now* … just as you told me *you want to feel completely safe*.

Doing things at high speed helps prevent the client from associating into the fear

Explanation of why they are doing these strange visualisations. (This should reinforce what you have told them pre-trance)

So that's why we're going to do that a few more times and each time we do it, we'll add in some other changes too … take a look at your remote control because you've got some other keys that you probably hadn't noticed before … so quickly get up the end safe scene on your mental screen … ready? … You're going to press the rewind and also press the size-change key and … hey … that's amazing … everybody except you shrinks down smaller and smaller … still speeding along backwards in that rather comical way … and let me know

Changing the size of characters or objects further breaks up the mental coding of the memory. Normally, the effect of reducing the size is also to reduce the fear attached to the situation. In addition, increasing the size of the self will often have an empowering effect. (Test this out as, very occasionally, this might not be the case *(continue on next page)*

11

when you get back to the opening scene where *you are totally safe and unconcerned* … quite nonchalant actually … look at your face … look at your body language … great job … now fill the screen with light … that's it, brighter and brighter so all you can see is wonderful bright light.

Now quickly get up that end scene again … that's it and this time … (what's your favourite song by the way? … OK. Great) … this time as you run the movie backwards … still really, really quickly … I'd like you to be singing your favourite song … really loudly … you can do it just in your head … (but actually there's no law against singing so you can sing out loud here and now if you want to) … whichever way you do it will be perfect for you but please do it really loudly and you can get the other people to join in too … let me know when you've done it and *you're safe and sound* at the beginning again. [Pause] Excellent. You *know what to do now* … let in the bright light again.

and then you would need to make other changes instead. If one of the fears centred around other people looking at them or feeling embarrassed, it would clearly not be appropriate)

Adding humour helps to reduce or remove fear and encourages the client to take things more light-heartedly

As mentioned before, this would not be appropriate when dealing with traumatic or tragic situations

- Each time the client rewinds the movie, stress the aspect of 'feeling calm and safe' on the opening and final scenes
- Repeat the procedure at least four or five times, making more changes to the speed (go more quickly), size, colour, sound, feelings, tastes and smells as appropriate with each rewind
- Have them turn everybody into cartoon characters or their favourite movie stars

Optional Insertion
After having carried out the rewind procedure on screen (dissociated), you can ask the client to mentally step into the film and imagine actually being there (associated) feeling themselves carrying everything out backwards. This is particularly good with people who have a strong kinaesthetic sense as it really helps to break up negative feelings.

Now this time I would like you to call up the opening scene of you looking exactly like your normal calm self … no funny colours … no different sizes … no cartoons this time … just looking perfectly relaxed and at ease and I want you to run the movie forwards, at normal speed, from start to finish and have yourself react coolly and calmly … just as you would have wanted to do … and when you get to the end and *you are feeling absolutely fine* … I want you to tell me what was different about it this time. [Pause]

Be prepared to repeat this procedure several times until the client is satisfied that their behaviour in the movie can't be improved in any way. You can also get them to run it through on fast forward several times to reinforce the new memory

Get feedback (If negative, reframe, give them extra resources, take them deeper, be prepared to add in different approaches)

So this time it felt better/you felt calmer/you felt more in control/you could even *see the funny side* … wonderful! … Could you *improve it* in any possible way? If so, just run it through in your mind with *you reacting even more calmly and confidently* … so you can *keep this memory in your mind* … which *is altogether easier for you*, is it not?

> While they are running through it again, you can add relevant direct suggestions for calm and confidence

And … the next/very last thing I want you to do is to *take a step into the screen* and *be there now* seeing things through your own eyes … and this time I want you to run a future movie of 'the calmer you' in a similar situation but noticing *how differently you handle everything now* … how you *feel confident inside* and how *you are completely in control of your feelings* … *you are completely in control of your actions* … let me know when you've finished and now tell me how *the experience was a whole lot different this time.* [Pause]

> Change from a dissociated experience into an associated one

> Presupposition of change

> Get feedback

Excellent … you have made some really life changing alterations to the way *you used to see/do things* and now I'm going to ask your unconscious mind to *make these new responses a very real part of your own inner world* … to fuse them into you so they *remain always with you* wherever you are … whomever you're with … whenever you're there and whatever you're doing. Now I think would be a good time for that observant part to float back into you and … I'm sure … you will agree with me on what an excellent piece of work you've done today and … although you and I know *how very different everything is going to be from now on* … have you been wondering how your husband/wife/son/daughter/ friend will react when they see you so calm and in control when you're on the bus/train? … Will you be looking at them with some amusement as they are looking at you wondering exactly what is going on?

> Not only alterations but 'life changing alterations'

> Reinforcement of the new inner responses

> Reintegration

> Presupposition of change

> Prepares the client for the fact that friends and family may be observing them and offers an 'amused reaction' to this.

Give more direct suggestions, more positive guided visualisation of a positive outcome or go directly to a trance reorientation as appropriate

Change anxious thoughts and images

And as you sit there, you can become aware of any possible stored tensions that you'd like to let go ... and ... just as soon as you're ready ... you can choose to *let them go with your breathing* ... and this may be the time ... when you need to *let yourself begin to find a way to rest right now* ... building your calm ... and *do know that you have that calm and confidence* deep down within you ... settling yourself down ... calm and confidence drifting up to the surface ... so I'd like you at first to *let only your eyelids rest* now ... letting every tiny little muscle and nerve ending rest and let go. Don't worry about the *rest* of you ... just concentrate on letting your eyelids rest ... that's right, making them more comfortable now. Let the feeling of comfort *spread right through the eyes, feel the comfort* and *know it's safe to enjoy those feelings of comfort now* ... and as you listen to the sound of the voice and as a calm feeling is beginning to come upon you ... so you can *begin to feel the comfort spreading* further ... and every place that it touches in your mind and body can *notice that comfort spreading calm* ... and now your eyelids are *really* resting, can you notice that different parts of your body are beginning to *feel more comfortable now*? And it's good to let them *feel even more comfortable now* ... all over ... all the way through.

And if you were to *become aware of any knotted feelings anywhere in the mind or body* ... imagine taking the knot in your fingers ... now find the loose end ... give it a little tug and notice how it loosens when *you pull it gently* ... how it unravels any old, unwanted anxious feelings ... how it seems to relax any unnecessary tension ... notice how it seems to *let every muscle go*, ease every tiny little muscle fibre ... *soothe every nerve ending in the mind and body* ... *wonderful.*

'and this may be the time' **is deliberately ambiguous as it relates both to the phrases before and after it**

Juxtaposition of 'settling down' **and** 'calm and confidence drifting up'

'let *only* your eyelids rest now' **eases fear of not being able to experience complete relaxation**

The word 'safe' **is reassuring and the sentence links ideas of safety, listening, calm and comfort together**

Now come the suggestions of calm spreading to other parts of the body

The metaphor of 'knots of tension' **is one often used in general speech and has good kinaesthetic appeal**

And even though you are aware of feeling this wonderful sense of relaxation, I wonder if you can *try* really hard to open your eyes ... that's right. Difficult, isn't it? ... But, well done [as their eyes open], you can just manage it ... I want you to know that ... in a moment ... when I ask you to let them close again ... there will be an experience of even deeper relaxation and calm ... for ... as your eyelids close ... they *release any possible remaining hint of tension* and you will *go into a profound state of calm and ease* where you can begin to understand things from a different perspective and find a way for you to *view your thoughts in a calmer way.*

Extemporise as appropriate to the response of your client. 'try really hard to open your eyes' suggests effort and some clients will struggle to open their eyes. However, others will open them easily for they have not, in truth, completely relaxed the eyelids yet. Either response is fine since the next suggestion is designed to relax them further

And if any intrusive/unwanted/anxious thought were to drift in ... don't fight it ... encourage it now and allow yourself to *listen to it in a more critical way* ... notice the tone of it ... notice the volume of it ... notice which direction it seems to come from ... and now begin to experiment with it and *become aware of the difference that each individual change creates in the way you respond* ... notice how *your body can feel differently too* ... make the inner voice louder ... make it quieter ... make it a high squeaky voice ... now a deep voice ... make it seem to come from the opposite direction ... get inventive! ... Keep the changes you prefer or simply reach out and turn the volume control off altogether.

You can choose whether to make this an interactive process, getting feedback from the client as you go along, or just to give open ended suggestions together with long pauses for experiment

Changing aspects of the inner voice can dramatically reduce an anxiety. It also empowers the client to see that they can take active control of a thought rather than be at its mercy

You may have noticed that an image accompanied the thought ... *take a mental step back and observe it fully* and notice the colours, the size, the position of it ... *become aware of any feelings that go alongside* and notice where they are in your body ... nod your head when you notice a colour ... that's it ... now let that colour fade away ... perhaps into a kind of sepia colour, just like a very old photograph ... nod your head when you've done it. ... Good, now send it away from you right over there ... further and further away so it becomes smaller and smaller ... and smaller still ... more and more insignificant now ... and I wonder if ... *you can, right now ... drain*

You may need to get them to experiment more with changing size, distance, position, colour etc. in order to achieve the desired effect. Be guided by your client

the colour completely away so it becomes quite transparent ... so you can see right through it ... see right through it for the fraud it used to be ... notice how it seems so much easier to *deal with it now ... calmly and coolly ...* coolly and calmly ... now white that thought out, white it out completely, calmly and peacefully now. Nod your head when that seems altogether more peaceful and calm ... Good job.

And so I think it will please you to know that you have gained a tool to *take control ... refuse to be intimidated* by old exaggerated thoughts ... *shrink them down into their genuine insignificance* so that you not only *stand up to those unwanted thoughts* but you *tower over them with your strength and calm and control.* And as you quite deliberately choose to let more and more *unhelpful thoughts fade into the distance in this way* ... you are going to find that they no longer have the power to affect you in that same old way ever again ... *you are the one with the power* to cut them down to size ... to *turn down the volume* ... to *switch off that inner voice* and replace it with one that is so much calmer and more rational.

Staying here just a little longer and *feeling a sense of satisfaction* with your own ability to *take control over old unwanted anxious thoughts* ... take a moment to notice how much more confident you can feel with this new ability to *calm your thoughts whenever* and *wherever* and *with whomever* you want ... think about how it can *seem so natural that you have much more control of your emotions.* ... It's also interesting, by the way, to consider *exactly how* you notice that *you are feeling much better already* ... do you feel lighter, as though a burden has been lifted off you, as indeed it has? ... Or would you describe it as a more grounded feeling? Well, whether you would use the words calmer, or lighter or grounded it's good to be aware that it is *your own mind* that has created this special state for you of peace and calm and confidence where your deeper, inner mind

> Use a strong, confident tone of voice to emphasize effect of the embedded commands and a sense of power

> The use of '*how* you notice' instead of *if* you notice presupposes that they are feeling better already

> You can also include expressions that they have used in your pre-induction talk

is released from old unwanted responses and can instead *be more and more open to new ways of responding calmly and confidently* here and now and then and sooner and later … each day learning more and more about your ability to *relax and enjoy your life in a calm and confident way.*

So, just before we finish today I think you would find it interesting to drift forward in your mind … as in a dream sequence … through the next few weeks and months and get a taste of just how positive it can feel to *experience this calm confident feeling as you go about your daily life* … so take a moment to … *dream now and look at the more confident you*, how you *feel so much calmer in your mind and in your chest, your tummy/your belly, your whole body* … altogether so much more relaxed … and hear, as well as see, how things are different now … *listen to your voice that sounds so much more assured* … yes … and also *your inner voice seems so much more rational and calm now* … and if ever there were to be the merest hint of an intrusive thought or image, you are now aware of how powerful it feels to be able to *change the effect of any thought or image in those proactive ways you learned with me* … and, of course … *the more often you practise* changing the colour, the size, the position of an image … or you practise changing the tone or the volume of an inner voice … *the more control you take* over those old outgrown thoughts so that they can *never disturb you in that same old way again.*

And as you bring all those insights from your new future back with you now and begin to reorient to your present surroundings … I find myself wondering whether it will be only you who is noticing these positive changes in you or whether your friends/family/partner will be noticing something very different too … and I wonder what is most enjoyable and what is most satisfying about all of this for you? … And for them? … And over the next few days and weeks

The implicit suggestion is that all of this will continue

'just before we finish' **alerts them to make the most of what is coming next**

Including personal references to the client's desired outcomes at this point will enrich the visualisation

Other people noticing a change reinforces the change itself

and months *there are going to be many things to notice and many things to enjoy.*

And you can even *enjoy an energising feeling at this very moment* ... rather as if you are awakening from a sleep/doze/nap which has refreshed and invigorated you ... eager to get on with your day ... a sense of calm purpose ... noticing that you want to stretch ... wriggle your fingers and toes. ... Welcome back!

Or use a more formal trance reorientation if appropriate

Fountain metaphor

The script includes the idea of standing in a fountain, so it is important to check that your patient does not have a fear of water.

So, relaxing comfortably here in the chair and becoming more and more aware of comfort spreading calm all around ... I wonder if you can begin to *imagine a feeling of mild warmth* ... maybe experiencing this warm feeling as though you could *feel the sun shining gently on your skin*? A lovely day with the temperature of the air just perfect for you ... and I wonder *how* you will imagine some special gardens ... perhaps beyond a gate, which you could *stroll through now into a very peaceful place* ... your own place where you can *be peaceful and calm* ... the grass is a vibrant green and gently springy beneath your step ... can you feel it? ... And when you look up, can you *notice how blue is the sky*? ... With occasional fluffy white clouds creating interesting patterns? ... And are there flower beds with wonderful colours and delicate fragrances on the air? ... Know that this is your own very special place that you can visit as often as you want to *let feelings of velvet calm come upon you* ... where others only enter at your special invitation ... so *pause awhile ... look around and breathe in the peace surrounding you* and ... as you stop and *listen now* ... you may seem to *hear the sounds of water* ... and walking down through the beds of flowers ... drawn towards that sound ... can you *catch a glimpse of a fountain in the distance*? The gentle rays of the sun still pleasantly warming your skin as you walk on towards the fountain ... coming closer now ... yes, standing right in front of it now ... so close that you can *extend your hand and feel the perfect temperature of the soft water on your skin* ... now moving closer and feeling a fine spray of water on your arms ... already *aware of a sense of letting go*

Your voice should be light and permissive as you set the scene and encourage active participation

Kinaesthetic
Visual

Deliberate phrasing of 'visit as often as you want to *let feelings*' **links one idea to the next**

Auditory

of tension ... becoming aware of an urge to *step into that fountain* and allow the water to spray over your entire body ... letting it flow over your face as it *washes away all remaining tensions* from the scalp ... from the back of your neck ... the water is washing away all unwanted anxieties from your shoulders, your chest, your stomach as it washes away all unwanted concerns from your mind ... feeling an immense sense of relief as the water now begins to cascade down ... cleansing, melting away sensations of tension, the body relaxes, the mind unwinds more and more comfortably ... bringing with it a crystal clear understanding ... that ... *this is the time ... this is the place ... this is your opportunity now* ... yes ... to *let go finally of any unwanted, unnecessary or harmful thought* ... that's it ... *let go any uncomfortable feeling* ... what a welcome relief ... *let go any long-outdated unhelpful response* ... from however long ago ... *let them all flow away* with the water ... at last ... what a weight off your shoulders ... and as the water cleanses you, watch the colour of it as it carries all that debris away ... splashing down into a little stream ... carrying it all away ... and you can keep watching until the water grows clearer and clearer ... and clearer still ... sparkling ... releasing you to *experience a delightful feeling of inner calm and confidence* ... a feeling of being at ease with yourself ... and when *you're at ease with yourself*, how much more natural it seems to *feel at ease with the world around you* ... staying here for a while allowing your imagination free rein to run through all those occasions in your life which *you will experience from now on with more calm ... with more courage ... with more curiosity ... and with more ease than you've done for a long, long time* or perhaps with more ease and confidence than you've ever done in your life before.

And when the time seems right to you to *move on*, nod your head and let me know. [Pause] Well done ... why don't you step out of the fountain now?

Adapt this section if you feel that your patient would not respond well to water flowing over the face. However, I have used this idea with countless patients and found that they all responded well

Include specific fears and anxieties mentioned by the client or keep it vague and all-embracing as appropriate. Be observant and leave pauses long enough for anxiety to be released

VK

Continue to observe and leave pauses throughout the whole section. Give more encouragement if required

… Yes, that's it … and find the sunlight instantly dries you, once again gently warming you … looking down at the now clear water of the stream and seeing your reflection sparkling back at you … look at your face … relaxed and smiling and at ease … one sparkling image replaces another … scene after scene of you feeling calm, confident and relaxed in those situations that you once used to feel uneasy about … now behaving in a comfortable and easy manner … allowing others as well as yourself to *feel that ease and calm* … in fact … so natural to you now that it can seem rather strange that it was ever not so. It does *seem so natural* that you have been able to *replace old concerned thoughts with those of calm and ease and confidence* … which now enable you to *go through your daily life with ease and equanimity.*

'the sunlight instantly dries you' **ensures they feel comfortably dry again**

Enrich this section with details of the patient's desired outcome in the specific situations discussed in the pre-induction talk

And as you begin to reorient to the room you can *enjoy this wonderful sense of ease and calm and confidence in your mind and in your body* that will stay with you as you *return to full conscious awareness of how calm and positive and optimistic you feel right now*. When you stretch … that's it … and open your eyes … you will *feel refreshed, revitalised and looking forward to a really positive day!*

Post-hypnotic suggestion for calm and confident feelings to remain post-trance

You may like to leave it here or go to a more formal trance reorientation if appropriate

Variations, Adaptations and Recommendations

This script could be adapted to form the basis of a framework for letting go of anger, frustration, guilt or grief. The use of water cleansing away unwanted, unhelpful emotion is a very powerful metaphor. Clearly, a means of coping with any original causes and/or any current triggers of these emotions would also need to be included.

Anxiety biofeedback

I wonder if you have you ever used a biofeedback machine where you rest your fingers on sensors and the sensors pick up physiological information through minute temperature changes and moisture on the skin? They can measure blood pressure, muscle tension and heart rate too ... absolutely amazing ... and even more amazing is that when you become aware of these things you can *gain control of these processes* in a way that allows you to *decrease levels of tension ... and increase your calm and relaxation* in a way you have never dreamed of before ... that's right ... *increase your calm and relaxation* in a way you have never dreamed of.

And some of these biofeedback machines are linked to screens where you carry out very simple tasks ... like slowing your breathing ... to *increase your calm and relaxation* ... and this calm and relaxation is then picked up from your fingers by the sensors and fed back to the screen where you see the result ... sometimes these are in the form of graphs ... sometimes they are through verbal feedback ... and sometimes they come in the form of visual images and interactive pictorial stories.

And ... as you really want to *get some relief* from the anxious thoughts and feelings that have been weighing you down ... I'd like to invite you to explore the biofeedback idea in your imagination with me right now so when you're ready to begin, please just nod your head ... excellent. In your mind's eye/imagination ... let your fingers rest on the sensors and look at the screen in front of you ... and you will see a gate ahead of you that will only open into the garden beyond when you *breathe calmly and deeply* and it senses *you are very calm and relaxed* ... let's try it now and see if it opens ... take a deep breath and inhale a sense of calm and comfort ... that's right ... and now with your out breath let go of any possible

Introduces the concept of biofeedback, and at the same time includes indirect embedded commands for calm and relaxation

Permissive suggestion which, when accepted, indicates willingness to take part in the imaginative task. Also note the presupposition of '*when* you're ready to begin' **rather than** '*if* you're ready'

22

tension ... and continue doing this until you are so calm and at ease that the sensors pick this up and the gate begins to open ... keep doing the breathing ... that's right ... breathe in the calm and breathe out the tension ... and let me know when the gate begins to open.

Leave plenty of time for the gate to open and you can use 'encouragers' such as 'that's right', 'well done', good job' **in time with their breathing**

[As you get a response] Excellent ... as you open the gate the whole garden is filled with a wonderful light and can you feel a sense of expectation as you walk through ... that something special is waiting for you here? An opportunity for you to *experience something interesting* that will *improve your life immeasurably*? Are you curious? The sensors will pick up the curiosity in your fingers and ... when they do ... you will be directed to a path for you to follow ... let me know when you notice the path. [Pause] Good ... so you're feeling curious ... let's see what happens.

Allow plenty of time

And as you walk along the path, I wonder if you are already sensing an opportunity coming closer ... to *free yourself of this burden/weight/millstone around your neck* that has been stopping you from moving forward in your life as quickly and easily as you would like? How long have you been carrying it around I wonder? Keep walking along and you will notice that the path opens out into a small clearing ... let me know when you notice the clearing.

Include any specific expression that the client has used to describe the 'burden' of anxiety

That's good ... walk along a little further and you will come to a rather lovely rock pool with a grassy patch around it where you could sit down for a while ... *enjoy the rest* for a few minutes ... enjoy just relaxing and breathing in the calm and the ease in this special place ... and once again, with your out breath ... breathing out the tension ... and I'm wondering if *it will be sooner* ... or a *little* later ... that the realisation begins to dawn on you that this is what your sense of expectation was about ... (funny how sometimes the most obvious things take a while to occur to us) ... and then when they do we can hardly believe how it's taken so long! ... Has it happened yet? That

Use your voice to encourage an air of gentle excitement

suddenly it's become clear that *you have a choice* ... you can decide here and now that *you really do want a better quality of life* ... one that is *not* ruled by persistent anxiety but one where *you are free to live your life in a satisfying and fulfilling way* ... in fact, of course ... you've already chosen to *take the first step* by entering this garden ... and when you are ready *to take the next step and shed the burden of those anxious thoughts and feelings* ... the sensors will pick this up from your fingers and cause your amazing unconscious mind to begin to seek out every unwanted, unhelpful, anxious thought or feeling ... *seek out the source* of every unwanted, outdated fear anywhere in your mind or body ... and you can *trust your unconscious mind to know just how to do it* ... and find a simple way for your conscious mind to *let the fear go here* in this garden.

So ... as all of this has been happening at the unconscious level ... have you already begun to *become more consciously aware* now how those thoughts and feelings seem to have transformed into heavy stones stored around your person/body ... perhaps in your pockets ... perhaps in a back pack ... but all within your grasp now ... so that you can actually pull/drag them out and place them on the grass ... some of them are very jagged and spiky aren't they? ... Some of them more like smooth pebbles that have been there a long time ... you can take a moment or two to think about the incredible difference it will make when you *say goodbye to anxiety* and *make space for calm and confidence in your life.* As you look at the different shapes and sizes of the stones can you recognise each one for what it really is? Which one is the fear of being judged/the unknown/losing control? ... Which one is the anxiety around taking responsibility/asserting yourself?

So now the time has finally come ... *your* time ... to *choose which one you want to drop into the rock pool first* and then really *enjoy heaving it into the*

Signals the idea that people can *choose* to exert control over anxiety and not simply be at the mercy of it

Encourages the client's acknowledgement that they have 'already chosen to take the first step'

Their conscious mind doesn't necessarily have to know how to do this as their unconscious mind will do it all for them

Use the information that you have elicited in your pre-induction talk rather than the examples given here

water and watching it sink to the bottom ... keep going until you have done all you need to do ... you can enjoy watching the water until every ripple disappears ... let me know when you are satisfied you've done all you need to do.

If by chance there were any left over ... you could always place them carefully under the bushes around the edge where they can *rest safely* ... where they can't disturb you ... where *they don't bother you at all* ... and if you so wish ... you could come back and *deal with them* at another time ... when you're ready ... but for now they can *rest safely there as you calmly get on with your life*.

How wonderful ... what an amazing relief that must be ... I think the sensors are picking up that relief from your fingers even as I speak ... let me know when you see a friendly figure coming towards you ... looks a bit like you actually ... with an air of seren-ity ... a sense of calm ... a lightness in his/her step ... it's the you from your future coming to guide you ... *support you* ... *give you strength* ... letting you know that *everything is going to be alright* ... eve-rything has turned out well ... he/she is guiding you down another little path towards a narrow, shallow stream where the water is clear and sparkling and ... as you come closer ... you can see there are step-ping stones that lead to the other side ... your com-panion is walking ahead ... crossing the stepping stones ... beckoning you to follow ... but you can pause awhile as you take all of this in ... as you look over to the other bank you realise that ... yes ... this is your future when *you want to take it* ... look at the 'future you' over there ... doing what you want to do ... look at your body language ... *easy and relaxed ... calm and confident now* ... listen to your strong confident voice as you meet and *deal with those challenges that you once used to avoid* ... how natu-ral you look ... taking things in your stride ... enjoy-ing taking those opportunities that you once *used to* shy away from. The figure is walking back towards

If you sense they have difficulty in letting all anxiety go, please include the following option

Optional Inclusion

This is a useful reserve position if they are unwilling or unable to release everything in one go

This metaphor contains the implicit presupposition that the client has been able to release their unwanted anxiety

Add in the client's specific, desired outcomes

25

you and waiting there on the other side of the stream and beckoning you to join him/her ... without that heavy weight it's going to be so much easier to cross now ... think about it ... and when the sensors pick up from your fingers that you do *really want to move into a happier, calmer, more confident future* ... you will see the 'future you' coming over to take your hand and help you over the stepping stones ... let me know when you see him/her.

Great ... a sense of excitement now ... stepping lightly yet firmly across ... feeling good ... make your way across to the other bank ... that's it ... it really is time for you to *enjoy being you ... enjoy spreading your wings ... notice a lighter feeling inside ...* stronger and more confident too ... and those *feelings of internal strength and confidence allow you to get on with living your life fully and naturally* ... with a whole range of responses appropriate to every situation ... very calm and relaxed ... or positively excited ...confident and in control ... comfortable with who and what you are. Well done/great job!

Go to a suitable trance reorientation

Hypno-desensitisation procedure

Read prior to using the desensitisation script.

1. Establish a hierarchy of the patient's feared situations using a Subjective Unit of Disturbance Scale (SUDS). Formally, this uses a scale from one to ten to measure the strength of fears experienced subjectively by the individual. You would elicit situations in your pre-trance discussion so they would produce something similar to the one below. You could also do this more informally and get them to list the fears they give you in order of their feelings of intensity rather than insisting on a one-to-ten scale.

Example of a SUDS of someone with a travel toilet phobia:

1. At home, merely thinking about going out	*very mildly nervous*
2. Walking to the station	*anxiety building*
3. On the platform, wondering if there will be a toilet in working order	*upset, anxiety building further*
4. Getting on the train and noticing how crowded it is	*anxiety becomes stronger, hot and upset*
5. Checking if there is a toilet	*feeling panicky*
6. Realising the toilet is occupied	*beginning to really panic*
7. Feeling sensations of needing to use the toilet	*beginning to 'freak out'*
8. Feeling of needing to get off the train before losing control	*strong panic, feeling it is unbearable*
9. Realisation they can't get off	*becoming hysterical, thinking they will break down*
10. Actually losing control of bowels on the train	*overwhelmed, feeling like a nervous breakdown*

2. Establish the new desired response.

3. Use a progressive relaxation induction and deepener.

4. Give direct suggestions for calm, safety and confidence.

5. Present the scenarios from the SUDS, beginning at the bottom of the hierarchy with the least threatening. The scene should show the patient handling the situation calmly and confidently (*Use the following Generic Template*).

6. Move to the next scene only when you have confirmation that they feel sufficiently calm to do so. You can ask them, get a head nod or finger lift (deliberate or an ideomotor response previously installed IMR).

7. Repeat deepening and direct suggestions for calm and confidence as required.

8. Continue to the top of the scale or to the point where the patient is comfortable. This can be done over one or more treatment sessions as required. Always make sure you end the session on a positive note. (Clearly in the above case, you wouldn't go to no. 10!)

9. Ego strengthening.

10. Trance reorientation.

Desensitisation of a phobic or panic response – generic template

This case uses the example of leaving the safety of the home and possibly using public transport. It would also be appropriate for many other presenting fears or anxieties. Replace shaded areas with suggestions appropriate to the particular phobia or situation.

In your pre-trance discussion it is essential to establish a hierarchy of fears.

Remember to respect the client's aims: it is not the therapist's place to insist that a client should, for example, pick up a spider unless this is a clear objective!

Use a progressive induction and a suitable deepener to induce as deep a trance as possible.

And feeling deeply calm and relaxed in this receptive state of hypnotic relaxation … just really *notice the sense of deep calm and relaxation you are feeling right at this moment* … nod your head when *you are aware of it* … good … I'm going to ask you to imagine some of the situations we spoke about earlier where you *used* to feel those unwanted panicky sensations so that now I can show you how you can *exchange those feelings for ones that are calmer and altogether more appropriate to you now at this stage in your life* … and there's no doubt that thinking and feeling and behaving calmly and confidently is far more appropriate for you … and … as you told me … *this is exactly what you want* … so from now on this is exactly what you are going to do … you are going to *think calmly and very confidently about* going out *whenever and wherever and however you want to* … you are going to *feel calm, comfortable and at ease* and you are going to *behave in a very natural, easy and ordinary way when* you're out

As you will already have elicited a hierarchy of fears, this will not come as a surprise

Direct positive suggestions reflect exactly what they want and concentrate the mind

Clients often say that they want to be 'normal/just like other people'

29

... just like other people do... no big deal ... your breathing will be regular and normal ... your heart will be beating regularly and normally ... your mind will be engaged in something more interesting ... in fact everything will be ordinary and normal in an everyday way ... so I'd like you to imagine in any way you like ... a screen in front of you ... it may be a television screen ... it may be a movie screen ... it may be a computer screen ... or it may simply be an awareness of a situation in your mind ... whichever way you become aware of this will be fine and it will be the most effective way for you.

Giving options allows freedom to imagine in their own way and so reduces any possible anxiety about needing to 'get it right'

Now bring up the first situation we discussed on that mental screen in front of you ... the one where you are at home just <u>thinking about going out</u> ... once again *be very aware of the sense of deep calm and relaxation you are feeling inside right at this moment* sitting in the chair in my consulting room/in my office ... and now breathe these calm steady feelings into the 'you' on the screen sitting/standing there ... and now watch that 'you' on the screen take a deep breath and *breathe in all the calm ... deep down inside* ... good that's right ... and notice how that 'you' is *handling the thought in a fairly ordinary/ matter-of-fact way ... born of a deep inner sense of calm* and a conviction that you really do want to *enjoy getting your life back ... being able to do the simple ordinary things in a very simple, straight- forward and ordinary way* ... you are calm ... look at your expression ... look at your body language ... nod your head when you can see it ... (or are aware of it in your own individual way) ... excellent ... so the next step is indeed a step ... I invite you to step into that scenario and *experience that calm thought and those ordinary comfortable feelings* just as though you are there ... you are there now ... nod your head when *you are right in the situation ... experiencing the thought in an ordinary comfortable way* ... good, that's right ... well done.

Present the lowest level in their previously established hierarchy of fears

They see the experience from a dissociated/ detached point of view

Now they experience it from an associated position

Now just step out of the scene for a moment while we have a look at the next one … feeling pleased with yourself and rather satisfied with how you are staying so calm as we do this … you can enjoy deepening your sense of calm even further as I count down from three to one … 3 … going deeper and deeper with each number you hear … 2 … that's it … and … 1 … feeling very calm, comfortable and relaxed … I would like you to be aware of the next situation that we discussed right there in front of you on the screen … the one where <u>you are walking down the road</u> … once again *be very aware of the sense of deep calm and relaxation … even deeper than before … that you are feeling right at this moment* … nod your head when *you are aware of it* … very good … now breathe those calm steady feelings into the 'you' on the screen just <u>walking down the road</u> in the most ordinary way and watch that 'you' take a deep breath and *breathe in all the calm feelings … deep down inside* … good that's right … and notice how <u>you are walking along</u> *in a fairly ordinary, matter-of-fact way … born of a deep inner sense of calm* and a conviction that you really do want to *enjoy getting your life back … being able to do the simple ordinary things in a very simple, straightforward and ordinary way* … look at your expression … look at your body language … notice that calm, steady relaxed breathing … nod your head when you can see that … or are aware of it in your own individual way … excellent … now once again I invite you to step into that scenario so you can *experience those calm ordinary everyday thoughts and those ordinary everyday comfortable feelings* just as though you were there … *you are there now* … nod your head when *you are aware of that sense of calm* … now listen to the very ordinariness/normality of the thought … <u>I'm going off to the station/I'm going to catch a bus/I'm going to pick up my child from school/I'm going to visit my friend, etc.</u> … Excellent … now when *you are very comfortable with that*, just nod your head and let me

The whole procedure is repeated with an extra 3–1 countdown deepener in preparation for each subsequent scenario in the hierarchy of fears. Additional suggestions for calm and confidence and extra deepeners can be added as required. The repetitious format for each scenario is useful since the client knows what to expect and any possible 'performance pressure' is removed. The suggestion for going deeper each time also deepens the trance state.

Dissociated

Associated

Once again, 'ordinary' or 'normal'

know. Excellent ... now just step out of the scene for a moment while we have a look at the next one.

So, wonderful ... feeling even more pleased with yourself and rather proud of how *you are staying so incredibly calm* as you do this ... you can enjoy deepening your sense of calm even more as I count down from three to one ... going deeper and deeper with each number you hear ... in fact, each time we do this you will *go even deeper than before* ... ready ... 3 ... deeper and deeper ... 2 ... deeper and deeper ...1 all the way deep down ... that's it ... and feeling very calm, comfortable and relaxed ... I would like you to be aware of the next situation we discussed right there on the mental screen in front of you ... the one where you are arriving at the station/ getting on the train/approaching the shops ... once again *be very aware of the sense of deep calm and relaxation ... even deeper than before ... you are feeling right at this moment* ... nod your head when *you are aware of it* ... very good ... now once again breathe those calm steady feelings into the 'you' on the screen just getting on the train/approaching the shops etc in the most ordinary way and watch that 'you' take a deep breath and *breathe in all the calm ... deep down inside* ... good that's right ... and notice how you are walking along *in a fairly ordinary/ matter-of-fact way born of a deep inner sense of calm* and a conviction that you really do want to *enjoy getting your life back ... being able to do the simple ordinary things in a very simple, straightfor- ward and ordinary way* ... look at your expression ... look at your body language ... notice that calm, steady relaxed breathing ... nod your head when you can see that ... or are aware of that in your own particular way ... excellent ... now once again I invite you to step into that scenario so you can *experi- ence those calm ordinary everyday thoughts and those ordinary everyday comfortable feelings* just as though you were there ... you are there now ... nod your head when *you are aware of that sense of calm* ... now listen to the very ordinariness of the thought

Only move on to each further step of the hierarchy after the client indicates that they are comfortable with the preceding one.

Embedded command which anchors deeper trance to the countdown

Dissociated

Associated

... 'I'm just getting on the train feeling perfectly OK/I'm going to visit my friend etc'. ... Excellent ... now when *you are very comfortable with that*, just nod your head and let me know. [Pause] Excellent ... now just step out of the scene for a moment while we have a look at the next one.

Repeat these steps until you have completed all the desired situations in the hierarchy with the client responding calmly. Only include appropriate situations as decided by the client. If necessary, you may complete this process in more than one session. If you do this, be sure to leave them feeling positive before terminating the session; deepen the trance and do a quick overview of the previous steps where they had experienced a calm and confident response. See the following Option One

Well, you've done some remarkably good work and I think it will very soon be time to complete the session for today with some extra calm and relaxation, so ... once again I'm going to count down from three to one and with each descending number you will become more deeply relaxed and calm ... ready ... 3 ... deeper and deeper ... 2 ... deeper and deeper ...1 all the way deep down ... that's it ... and feeling very calm, comfortable and relaxed ... that's it ... with each in breath breathing in the calm and with each out breath breathing out any hint of tension ... that's it ... I'd just like to remind you of how well you've done today and the excellent progress you have made ... you managed to think very calmly about the prospect of going out ... and you were able to walk to the station in a very ordinary, matter-of-fact way ... and you calmly waited on the platform and then got on the train and travelled a couple of stations [as appropriate]. Perhaps you can just run through that very, very quickly in your mind ... as if on fast forward ... and be very proud of yourself for what you have achieved today ... and when you have finished ... just let me know so that I can gently begin to help you reorient to the room. [Pause] Excellent ... I want you to know that with each day that passes *your unconscious mind will be strengthening your new responses* ... you will *find yourself drawn to carry them out and reinforce the ease with which you do them* so that by the time we meet next time *you will be feeling even more calm*

Option One
Early curtailment of the session

Deepen the trance

Congratulations on progress creates a sense of achievement and positivity

and confident … each day you will feel drawn to carry out your self-hypnosis/listen to the CD/do your positive thinking and feel stronger and calmer and more confident … not only about <u>travelling</u> but in so many other areas of your life.

Strengthens the desire to carry out the self-hypnosis homework to reinforce work done in the session

Go to a suitable trance reorientation

Wonderful … now you've managed all those steps with a calm and confidence you should be proud of … I'd like to invite you to run through the whole scenario as though watching a movie … and as it's your own movie with you in the lead role … make it the calmest, most confident one you can imagine … see it through exactly as you want it to happen and let me know when you've done it. [Pause] Well done … just think about it for a moment and if there is any possible way in which you could improve it, just run it through again adding in all possible improvements and let me know when you've done it. [Pause] Excellent … so now this is your memory and you can *keep this memory in your mind* … running through it as often as you like to reinforce it if you want to … so that from now on *this is how things will happen* … this is how your mind is programmed to *repeat this habit of calm and confidence* … it is deeply embedded in you now … as the days and weeks go past it will become just like any other good habit where you don't even have to think about it … you *just do it without even thinking about it* … so it's safe to forget about any old outgrown unwanted ways of doing things almost as if they never existed … never existed at all.

Option Two
Run through a calm and confident overview of all the steps on the hierarchy. Then invite them to keep improving it until it couldn't possibly be any better

Go to a suitable trance reorientation

34

Variations, Adaptations and Recommendations

Causes of anxiety may be many and various and may need to be addressed separately in different ways, for example cognitive restructuring, rewind procedures, parts work, regression plus cathartic release and insight, both instead of and as well as desensitisation. However, calm induced through desensitisation alone will frequently generalise and neutralise fears.

The desensitisation procedure and script can easily be adapted to treat most different fears and situations, as can the script *Let go of panic* which is a helpful script to reinforce other approaches.

Other useful techniques to make use of are the neutralisation of negative anchors and the installation of positive ones.

Fear of flying and desensitisation

Fear of flying can be very well treated using a desensitisation procedure. Common times of anxiety, feared scenario and panic triggers include:

- The days or weeks leading up to a flight, particularly when alone, unoccupied or at night
- Booking a flight
- Packing
- The journey to the airport
- Check-in procedures
- Super vigilant search procedures
- Going to the gate prior to departure
- Boarding the plane
- Fastening seat belts
- Closing of the doors (major trigger)
- Preparing for take-off
- Take-off and ascent with all accompanying sounds and sensations
- Turbulence
- Changes in engine tone
- Chimes
- Announcements
- Fasten seat belt signs
- Not being allowed to use the toilets
- Bad weather conditions
- Anything which could be perceived as unusual
- Announcement of pre-landing procedure
- Descent and landing with accompanying sounds and sensations.

The causes include:

- A sense of having no control over the aircraft or their destiny
- A fear of losing control and becoming hysterical
- A sense that, compared to other transport accidents, there is a greater chance of fatalities
- An overestimated sense of the risk involved
- Lack of understanding of basic principles, for example the plane is too heavy to stay in the air
- Previous frightening flight experience

- News of any air disasters, near disasters or terrorist activity prior to the flight
- Having children often initiates a great need in mothers to protect offspring from danger and people who have flown quite happily until then can become very frightened of flying
- Previous flights made to visit ill or dying relatives can cause fearful associations between flying and death.

Useful anchors:

- Physical anchors: gestures, fastening seat belts
- Visual anchors: the seat in front, the steward's face, looking out of the window
- Auditory anchors: chimes.

Let go of panic/anxiety

This script is intended for use as reinforcement, *having previously carried out a rewind or a desensitisation procedure.* A progressive relaxation would be an ideal induction.

Using a very rhythmic delivery within a stream-of-consciousness approach works well with this script which has within it much intentional repetition and linking of relaxation with acceptance of suggestions.

Sitting comfortably there ... just listening and relaxing and accepting positive suggestions that will help you ex*change that old panicky way of responding for a calm and comfortable response* ... you can enjoy taking on an overall sense of controlled well-being now you have made the decision to *let go of that old unhelpful reaction* ... and because you have already made that decision to welcome suggestions for calm and controlled well-being ... your unconscious mind has been becoming more and more open and receptive and all you need to do is to *enjoy just listening and relaxing and accepting the positive suggestions* that we discussed before ... and as you *go deeper and deeper* you *enjoy just listening and relaxing even more* ... knowing this is the right thing for you ... just enjoying accepting the positive suggestions that you have agreed will *improve your life immeasurably* ... just listening and relaxing ... that's it ... just listening and relaxing and accepting that this is what *you truly want* as you *go deeper and deeper relaxed* ... hearing *my voice calming and relaxing you with every word and each suggestion you accept* ... as you *go deeper and deeper* ... just listening and *enjoying accepting* ... *feeling yourself accepting* that at last *you are changing things to your advantage* ... it's something you've wanted for so long and *now you can have it* ... it's yours as you *go into the deepest trance you've ever dreamed of* ... knowing now there is no going back on your decision to *let go of panic and being so grateful for that* ... accepting more and more ... almost completely in

The presupposition 'you have made the decision' is followed by the **embedded command** 'to *let go of that old unhelpful reaction*'

Reminder of what has been agreed in the pre-trance discussion

Sounds like a long awaited gift to be accepted

that receptive state now as you listen …. just listening and accepting the ideas and becoming more and more completely relaxed … so *completely sure you are doing the right thing* … so deep and accepting … hearing and *feeling the truth of my voice now* … feel my words that you *can't wait to accept them* … you *feel drawn to follow them* … and because you can't wait to accept them … you *feel compelled to follow them … following every word … following every single step of the way* … you're going to find that the old overstimulated responses/behaviour is starting to *drift away from your mind as you go deeper and deeper … drift away from your body* as you *go deeper and deeper … drift away from your very being all together* as you continue going deeper and deeper … you are more and more sure that the old thinking … the old behaviour has been drifting further and further away as though *it has nothing to do with you now* … no longer a part of you … almost as though *it was never there* and it will *become more and more difficult … to* bring it to mind no matter how hard you might try … and the harder you tried to think about it or recreate it …. the more difficult … the more impossible it would become … in truth *you are delighted that the feeling of calm confidence is becoming more and more what you want for you* … just enjoying listening and relaxing and accepting that the calm and confidence is settling down into you … embedding itself into you … it is now a part of you … it's what you really want … as each day passes it is becoming more and more part of your own inner way of *thinking calmly* … more and more part of your own inner way of *breathing calmly* … inner level and outer level … more and more part of you … your confidence is growing daily … here and now as *you are going deeper and deeper still … your belief in you is settling in deeper and deeper … growing stronger and stronger* … your belief in your confidence and your ability to *do things calmly and confidently* is growing stronger and stronger … the old response has been disappearing and *you are feeling more and more at one with your*

Very compelling

'over stimulated responses/behaviour' **is a reframe of panic**

The law of reverse effect

'embedding itself into you' **If something is 'embedded' it is difficult to dislodge**

'settling in deeper and deeper' **Once again, this seems difficult to dislodge**

calm way which suits you better ... *more and more comfortable and at ease* with it ... *more and more confident and comfortable* in the calm confidence being part of you ... in fact so comfortable and so confident that it hardly seems like a new way at all ... it just seems to be what you do ... you love being 'this you' with this calm, relaxed way of doing things ... *it's so right for you* ... you find *you are thinking calmly and confidently* ... happy and content in the way you do things now ... knowing that everything seems right now ... more appropriate now ... more 'you' now ... you keep the changes now at the inner level and they show automatically at the outer level and all the way through ... you *think calmly and confidently* ... you *feel calm and confident* and so quite naturally you *behave calmly and confidently* in everything that you do.

With the calm and confidence firmly embedded within you ... you will find that from now on *you will be responding naturally calmly in whatever you do* ... naturally confidently wherever you are ... naturally cool calm and collected in your thoughts both when you are alone and when you are with other people ... you *have a sense of being calm and steady/ well grounded/centred in your body as well as in your mind* ... with everyday that passes *this calm response is growing stronger and stronger* so that ... as the days turn into weeks and the weeks turn into months ... there comes a time when it seems strange for you not to *believe this strength and calm has always been there ... it has always been there ...* so now ... can you notice that standing before you is the 'you' who's *already absorbed all these sugges-tions ... made all the changes* ... just look at her in your mind's eye and with some delight/pride take a look at her body language so calm and relaxed as she is walking around the supermarket/walking into the interview/driving down the motorway/highway ... notice how she is breathing regularly and naturally ... all the systems of her body responding regularly and naturally ... clearly her mind is fully focused

'which suits you better' **carries the implication that a sense of calm is natural to the person**

In this next section the pronouns 'she' or 'her' have been used purely to avoid clumsiness in the script. Adapt as appropriate

Personalise this guided visualization of a successful outcome using information elicited from the client

on <u>the shopping/the driving/the conversation/the task in hand</u> … handling anything and everything … both expected and unexpected remarkably well … see how she is taking everything in her stride … well done … great job … and as you look now and see how *things have turned out so well* … it's right that you congratulate yourself for having had the foresight to *know just what to do and how to do it so effectively.*

Go to a suitable trance reorientation

Includes a positive embedded command for the present within the context of an imagined positive outcome

Travel toilet phobia

The mode of transport referred to here is the train but clearly the script can be adapted for use with any other form of transport. The script deals with commuting to work but it can easily be adapted for other travel experiences. Read it through carefully before use to see where and how it may be adapted. Depending on the severity of the phobia, it can be used as stand alone or in conjunction with desensitisation, rewind procedures or other approaches.

You have explained some of the difficulties that obsessive fearful thoughts and feelings about needing to use the toilet/bathroom/rest room while travelling has caused you over the months/years and, you, of course, know better than anyone else how this way of thinking has been shrinking your world ... depriving you of enjoyable experiences as time has gone by ... so of course, by the same token, ... you *know better than anyone else the differences that this experience today will make* to the enjoyment of your life ... that your decision to come here today will *start an ongoing process* of *taking your life back* into your own hands and extending possibilities ... creating opportunities for *going about your daily life in a calm and confident way* where your thoughts will *change their focus onto something altogether more enjoyable and interesting* ... so as you simply just relax comfortably there and drift and dream a little ... one of the things I'd like you to discover today is what will *be the very best thing for you about having made those changes* ... yes ... so many things to choose from.

Lets the client know you have been listening, validates them as the 'expert' on themselves but also emphasizes the idea of a shrinking and deprived experience of life. This should reinforce the desire to change

Note the embedded commands throughout

Gives them the opportunity to focus internally on the positive effects of behaviour change as against their usual negative orientation

Now you have told me that, in fact, ... despite all your conscious anxieties to the contrary ... *you have always been able to retain ultimate bodily control* ... even when it was difficult ... *you have always been able to stay in control* ... so it's good to know that your unconscious mind, that regulates the systems of your body, *can hold on very well even under quite difficult circumstances* ... so it's a relief to know that

Optional Inclusion
Only use where you have been assured that the client has never actually lost control of bowel or bladder function in the feared situations

your body knows how to do this at the unconscious level … so your task today is to get your body to *reassure your mind that it is perfectly capable of doing its work* and then your mind can allow your body to carry out its task more comfortably … more calmly … *keep your tummy/stomach/belly/bowel/ gut calm and comfortable* … so you *feel a sense of comfort and calm all over and all the way through*.

The wording allows reframing and embedding of commands

Relaxing more comfortably and deeply and really enjoying this experience of physical relaxation … it's good to know that you don't even have to *know consciously how* your mind and body will *experience a deep sense of calm reassurance* … it can all happen at the unconscious level … as you are relaxing even more comfortably … for your mind is expanding its horizons … and will automatically *take on the suggestions which will calm and relax every cell … every atom of your mind and body* … it can take in these suggestions through your breathing now … take them right deep inside your body … so breathe in these thoughts very deeply now … 'your stomach/bowel is safe … it can *stay calm and comfortable* … it can *stay calm and steady* … it will *hold onto its contents … hold on* until the time and place that you choose to allow them to empty … that's it … breathe very deeply … your stomach/bowel is safe … you are safe … now this knowledge is comfortably embedded deep within your body … every part of you knows they are completely safe … both your mind and body are calm and relaxed so they work in wonderful steady, gentle harmony together … wonderful … well done.

Embedded commands follow the phrase 'you don't even have to'

Being told 'it can all happen at the unconscious level' **removes pressure**

Breathing the suggestions directly into the gut allows them to settle into the right place

Excellent … now that *all of this is understood* and the knowledge is stored in your stomach/gut … you can allow your conscious mind to *forget all about it* … no need to bother about it at all now. From now on you will find that when you wake in the morning *you will wake refreshed after a good night's sleep* … you will use the bathroom in a calm and relaxed way and your stomach/tummy will feel comfortable and

Presupposition of understanding and stored knowledge

at ease … your mind will be focusing on your work/ your day ahead/whatever pleasant thing you like … as you drive/walk to the station, you will be gently aware that something is rather different but not quite sure what it is … just noticing things around you in a more enjoyable/appreciative way … somehow faintly aware that there is an optimism in the air … (or is it in you?) … even if it is cloudy or raining or chilly, there is a feeling of gentle buoyancy in you that you really rather like … interesting that you can *experience calm and buoyancy at the same time* is it not? … When you arrive at the train station … you make your way calmly onto the platform and await your train *with an equanimity* that may vaguely surprise you in a pleasant sort of a way … your thoughts keep drifting on to a pleasing and absorbing thought … which produces wonderful mental and physical feelings of calm and comfort … even when people around you may be pushing and jostling for position … when the train arrives you simply get on it and find a seat … or *stand calmly if there isn't one available* … you seem to *feel as though you are surrounded by an invisible bubble of calm and relaxation* which protects you from anything and anybody … it protects you from any formerly unwelcome thought since anything unwanted would merely rebound off the protective bubble barrier surrounding you … you will find that … now your unconscious mind has taken responsibility for keeping *you feeling calm and safe* … your thoughts will have taken on an outward focus and you are no longer as interested in your internal well-being … you are fully absorbed in your book/paper … and since your body is calm and relaxed inside you're scarcely consciously aware of yourself at all … just aware that your unconscious mind has everything under control *in the best and most calming way* so that … whatever may be going on around you … wherever you are … whenever you're there … whomever you're with … your stomach/bowel is content to *feel safe … feel relaxed … feel calm … feel soothed and steady inside.*

Personalize this guided visualisation with aspects of a journey as previously described to you

Use a pre-arranged pleasant thought for the client to focus on and trigger thoughts and feelings of calm

'Safe' is a very calming word

Repetition of the word 'safe'

As the days and the weeks and the months go by … because your unconscious has decided to *let go of that old outdated way of thinking* … and *because* you are able to *relax far more at a deep inner level now* … you will find that travelling anywhere any time is becoming just something that *happens as a normal part of your routine* … you are able to consign old responses to the past … *it's safe to forget about it more and more completely at the conscious level* … safe in the knowledge that your body has stored the calm and steady feelings of safety and gentle natural control at the inner level deep down inside.

Repetition of the word 'safe'

Allow your mind to travel forward to that time when things have normalised … that's it … *enjoy that feeling … a calm and comfortable composure with a lightness of heart* … and now turn around and look back to the time when those changes started to occur … did they happen gradually over time or did they begin to *improve quite dramatically*? Have a good look and notice just how many amazing changes have taken place. Look at the calm and composed body language … your mind is totally absorbed in your book/paper to *the exclusion of almost everything and everybody* around you … check in on those easy internal thoughts … notice how … whether the car/carriage is empty or crowded … seems to have no relevance at all … you look so light hearted, do you not? Wonderful … take as long as you want to enjoy this and once *you are ready to bring the experience of change and all those positive feelings back with you to the present moment of (today's date)*, just nod your head and I will help you reorient to the room.

Go to a suitable trance reorientation

Travel toilet phobia and desensitisation suggestions

Travel toilet phobia can also be very well treated using a desensiti-sation procedure. The following list contains a selection of sugges-tions for use within such a procedure:

- Your stomach/bowel/body is safe ... it can stay steady and comfortable.
- Your stomach is safe and you are safe.
- Your body will stay calm and comfortable throughout the journey.
- Your bowel/gut will hold onto its contents until the time and place that you choose to allow them to empty otherwise they will hold on.
- They will only empty at the time and place of your choosing.
- Now this knowledge of calm comfort is comfortably embed-ded in your stomach/gut ... your body knows it is completely safe.
- Both your mind and body are calm and relaxed so they work in wonderful steady, gentle harmony together.
- Your mind is outwardly focused.
- You're hardly aware of your body at all.
- You are calm, comfortable and composed.
- The harder you were to try to focus inwardly the more your thoughts would drift onto something else entirely.
- The harder you would try to think about yourself the more dif-ficult that would become as your thoughts seem compelled to drift onto x (an agreed pleasant topic).
- Whether the train is crowded/full or empty seems irrelevant to you now.
- Other people don't bother you at all.
- Whether the train has a toilet/restroom seems irrelevant to you.
- You feel mentally and physically confident and at ease as you travel.

Anchors – Explanation and Procedure

Anchors are essentially powerful triggers for a behavioural response which is associated with something already experienced. They can be positive or negative: negative, as in the case of seeing a syringe, smelling the antiseptic and immediately feeling faint; positive as in the case of hearing a snatch of 'your song' and being put into a good mood because it transports you to a wonderful time from long ago. Anchors come in all kinds of shapes and sizes; something you see, hear, feel, smell or taste can cause an instant reaction.

In real life these anchors are accidental; they just happen and we respond to them naturally. But in hypnotherapy we deliberately aim to take the power away from negative anchors which underlie many fears and phobias and, conversely, we aim to empower people by giving them positive anchors to trigger resourceful states. Sometimes it can be merely reminding them of a special achievement they felt proud of or a situation where they felt very calm and confident in order to allow them to reaccess that feeling in the moment, but other times it can involve a more structured approach to give them a gesture, a thought, or a phrase which they can reproduce at will to trigger a resource state whenever they need it. The *Anchors generic script* makes use of anchors, but you can use the procedure below both in or outside of a formal trance state.

Setting an anchor

1. Decide which trigger you will use – perhaps squeezing the finger and thumb together, squeezing your fist or taking a deep breath. It could be a phrase or a mental image that you can call immediately to mind. It needs to be something which can be remembered and reproduced exactly. It should preferably be unobtrusive so that other people will not notice what is being done.

2. Decide which resource state is appropriate to be triggered, for example confidence/calm.

3. Close your eyes and think of a time when you remember feeling particularly confident/calm. Let yourself remember exactly what that felt like and experience it all over again in your mind. Bring back the feelings, remember what you could see around you and see that picture in your mind again, maybe remembering what you were hearing at the time and fully imagine it happening to you right now. As the memory and the experience get stronger, set the chosen trigger, for example squeeze your finger and thumb together, and capture the feeling in your fingers as you link it with the remembered experience. You can also see the same picture in your mind's eye and say a word or phrase to yourself at the same time, for example Calm/Stay cool/Go for it!

4. Open your eyes and let the gesture go before the positive feeling begins to fade. You want to keep the link as strong as you can.

5. Repeat steps 3 and 4 three times.

6. Test the anchor. Make the gesture or take a deep breath, say the word or phrase to yourself, see that picture in your mind and notice how it brings back that positive feeling. If it fails to do so or isn't strong enough, repeat steps 3 and 4 until it works.

7. Once you have tested it and found it works you can rehearse using the anchor in the situation where you want to feel confident or calm or whichever other resourceful state you want. Do a guided visualisation and practise firing the anchor as many times as you can so it strengthens the anchor for use in the real world whenever it is required.

8. Use the anchor often; frequent use will strengthen not weaken it.

Confidence anchor – generic script

This particular script uses confidence as a resource, but it is generic in the sense that you can substitute any resource state desired by the client. It can be used as a stand-alone script or incorporated into almost any other script you choose to use.

It is useful to run through the procedure with the client beforehand so they know what to expect and to have a little time to think of an appropriate reference experience for setting the anchor.

And relaxing so comfortably there in the chair … just enjoying the thought that … as you *become deeper and deeper relaxed* … you are allowing your unconscious mind to do something today that will *improve the quality of your life* in so many ways … you explained that a major improvement in your life will be to <u>speak/perform/teach</u> *calmly and confidently* … with this calm and confidence springing from an inner belief in yourself.

Restates objectives and also embeds suggestions for calm and confidence

So it's good to know that your unconscious mind is a little bit like a safe/special box that holds all your valuables/jewels but in this case … the valuables/jewels are your inner strengths and all your positive memories too … now here's the particularly wonderful thing … in just a moment, we can turn these strengths and positive memories into powerful instant resources so that they can *be there at your disposal* … any *time* you want them … any *place* you want them … and with *anyone* that you want to use them so (as I explained to you earlier) the first thing you need to do is to *think of a time or situation where you were very, very confident* and … in a good way … very self assured … so open your box/safe and find something special … a really *positive confident memory* and allow yourself to *drift off to that time and place and be there now in the centre*

49

of this memory right now and *enjoy again this inner sense of confidence and belief in yourself* … noticing what you see and hear around you … and when *this awareness of confidence is really strong* … *capture this confidence between your finger and thumb* … (just the same finger and thumb gesture that we decided on earlier) and you can even *intensify this* by giving yourself a really powerful message right now. [Pause] Well done/good job … and now you can relax the fingers and let them part before this wonderful feeling could even begin to fade.

With your client's permission, enhance this response by touching them on the shoulder (or hand) with reasonable pressure at exactly the same time as they make the finger and thumb gesture. Release the pressure as they release their fingers *before the confident feeling begins to fade*

Very well done indeed … now let's strengthen the power of this gesture … (which will become your trigger for confidence) … by repeating this a couple of times in a moment … each time intensifying the image in your mind … intensifying the positive feeling in your body … intensifying the positive message in your head and strengthening the effect of the gesture … so once again … *be there now in the centre of this memory*, etc., etc.

Repeat two or three times until the association is really strong

Good … now just for a moment think about something entirely different, such as your journey home, just to distract yourself … or even open your eyes. [Pause] Now allow them to close again … and make that same gesture as before with your finger and thumb and *notice what happens … notice what image springs instantly to mind* … notice what feeling comes into your body and notice what *positive thoughts come to mind* … tell me what you experience. [Pause] [Assuming it is the confident response] Excellent … this is your trigger for extra confidence wherever … whenever … and with whomever you want it … all you have to do is to squeeze your finger and thumb together when you want to *deal with a situation more confidently* and you will *experience an extra surge of confidence all over* … in your mind … in your body and even *your voice will experience it strongly and steadily*.

They need to break the positive state so that they can test the anchor to check that it does indeed trigger the desired state
Be sure that they are reproducing the same gesture and not changing fingers!

Strengthen it/add in extra resources states if necessary

Now let's run through a few scenarios in detail in your imagination where you want some extra confidence … use your finger and thumb trigger at just the right moment … and enjoy the positive effects. [Long pause] Well done.

Do a personalised guided visualisation with the client having a positive outcome through using the anchor.

I wonder whether you have any idea yet when and where you will first *use the trigger once you leave here* … will it be *in one of those situations you told me about* or will it be something quite different? … You'll probably find it interesting … or even amusing … to discover all kinds of situations where it will be helpful … to *have that surge of confidence that lets you handle everything so* very positively … and actually there's another benefit too … think of the effect of having that *reassuring inner security that constantly accompanies you now you have your own personal confidence trigger* … Great job/well done.

Go to a suitable trance reorientation or continue with another script

Mild to Moderate Depression

These scripts are suitable for patients who are mildly or moderately depressed. I recommend Michael Yapko's work (1992 and 2001). His discussion regarding the treatment of depression is invaluable.

Treating patients who are depressed

- Pace the patient sufficiently for them to feel understood otherwise there will be no progress. It is important, however, not to get drawn into their negative trance story.
- They may have told this story many times and each time they tell it, the depression gets reinforced, so break it up with questions which are future- and solution-focused.
- Lead them towards their own solutions so they can invest in them. This is important because solutions proffered by the therapist may result in 'Yes, but ...' or 'I've tried it and it doesn't work.'
- Focus on things which they can change rather than on situations (or people) that are difficult or impossible to change.
- Encourage them out of feelings of helplessness into responsibility for change, however small.
- Don't overdo the positivity or they will be overwhelmed and not attempt any change.
- Use forward looking approaches not ones that reinforce depression by going over and over past hurts, rejections and misery. Solution Focused and Cognitive Behaviour Therapy (CBT) approaches have a good track record in treating depression.
- Collaborate with your client. Agree on small steps for specific achievable goals or they will become overwhelmed and even more depressed when they are not achieved.
- People who are depressed spend much of their time immersed in negative thoughts and feelings and their downward focus eye position seems to reinforce this. It is useful to encourage them to physically look up where their natural eye position may encourage visualisation. Encourage them to focus on small achievements with tangible results.

Depression: considerations and aims

An understanding of state dependent memory illustrates how we are more likely to recall memories reminiscent of the state we are currently in, i.e. when we are already in a negative and depressed state we likely remember negative memories and find it difficult to recall happy times. This is borne out in the therapy room where patients will frequently say their week was completely miserable, although specific questioning can often reveal that there were occasions where they actually enjoyed themselves or at the very least were not totally miserable. It isn't the case that there are not good times, it is that they are genuinely difficult to recall. In the trance state it is useful to give post-hypnotic suggestions to remember specifically pleasant or happy occasions they encounter.

If patients are highly medicated they may well sleep during the trance state if they become over-relaxed, and in any case they will already be in an altered state of awareness. Use inductions which are light, probably just conversational, and encourage focus rather than deep relaxation.

Suitable aims

Encourage them to:

- feel less helpless
- be more hopeful and realise that things can change for the better
- become more aware of how small specific practical steps can positively affect a situation
- become aware of things they are managing to do better than they thought
- become aware of their own internal resource states, past and present
- understand how they can make use of these resource states now and in the future
- build stronger resource states
- recall pleasant occasions, stronger thoughts and feelings that they have experienced in both the more distant and very recent past
- do something active, for example go for a walk
- have contact with other people.

Discovery

This script makes use of dissociation to allow a different perspective on current thoughts and behaviour in order to discover which patterns are unhelpful and which ones can move the patient forward. Dissociation can induce trance very quickly so this script may be used either with or without a formal induction.

In order to avoid clumsiness in the script I have used feminine pronouns.

You've told me a lot about how things haven't gone right and how sad/depressed/miserable/dejected/hopeless you have been feeling … you've told me how you've tried many things that haven't seemed to … *help you a great deal* … and you've also told me that you feel overwhelmed and that you haven't really known which way to turn to *find your way through this*.

> This paces their thoughts and feelings and shows you have been listening. Adapt it as appropriate to reflect your client's words
>
> Includes embedded commands

And yet … despite all of that … you have come to see me because *you do want to find a way through this and come out the other side* … so, well done for that … I'd like to invite you now to *take a break … through* the hypnotic state of hypnotic relaxation where you can *see things a little bit differently* … where *some aspects* can *become a little bit clearer than before* … where *you can appreciate how you handle some things rather better than you thought* … and begin to *discover how you can increase your ability to cope* while you are finding your way through (the tunnel) and out the other side.

> Use your voice to subtly link and emphasise the words 'break … through' to encourage unconscious acceptance of the idea of a 'breakthrough'
>
> Orients the focus onto the idea of increasing coping skills
>
> Omit 'the tunnel' if there are claustrophobic issues

So, taking a moment now to allow yourself a chance to *relax a little* … some people just *relax a little* and some people *relax a lot* … and some people **first** *relax a little* and **then** *relax a lot* … and of course the way *you* do it will be the perfect way for you … and as you are sitting there with your eyes closed, I'd like you to think about all the tiny little muscles and nerve endings in your eyelids … hundreds of them just in your eyelids … and let them relax [Pause] then double the relaxation … becoming aware now of the

> Permissive suggestions

comfort spreading right into the eyes … underneath the eyes … above the eyes … and does it spread down into the cheeks and into the jaw before it spreads up into the forehead and into the scalp … or is the other way around? Does it seem to spread from the scalp and the forehead down to the cheeks and the jaw? Well, whichever way it occurs … you can just let it happen and allow the comfort to begin spreading around your body as you continue to listen to my voice … and that easy, pleasant, comforting feeling can continue to spread all over your body … all the way through this experience of relaxation.

And now … as your body just rests comfortably there … allow yourself to imagine that you can experience the more observant part of yourself floating up above you … high enough above you for you to be able to observe yourself sitting there relaxing so comfortably … and let me know when you're there. [Pause] Thank you … and now have a look at [Client's Name] and just notice how she is coping with things in her everyday life. I'm going to suggest one or two things, Observant Part, for you to look out for … and you can, of course, choose whether you want to consider these things mentally and silently to yourself or whether you want to tell me what you notice … it's entirely up to you. … So from that bird's eye view … perhaps you can *notice some of the things that [Client's Name] is doing rather better than she gives herself credit for?* … From up there you may *notice that she has been finding and using an inner strength* which has enabled her to *persevere* even when things have seemed very difficult … notice some of the things that are working out not too badly … in fact … really … reasonably well. [Pause] And now have a think about what small changes she could make so that things work out a bit better still.

Good. What I'd like you, Observant Part, to do now is to float right over there to [Client's Name]'s left and take a seat … so that you can get a different per-

Allow the patient to choose whether to do all of this internally or to interact with you. If they choose to tell you their thoughts and observations, you will need to take them into account and extemporize but you can still use the script as a loose framework or guideline

Depressed patients may reject suggestions that seem over optimistic or too far outside their comfort zone. Suggestions such as 'rather better', 'not too bad', 'reasonably well' **will likely be better accepted**

spective on what needs to be done. ... What do you think is the smallest step she could take that would make a difference to the situation which would *allow a more positive outlook* ... allow a more positive outcome? ... And I wonder what would follow as a consequence when she takes that small step?

What if ... the negative 'what ifs' could be changed to more positive 'what if's'? I wonder if you, Observant Part ... sitting beside [Client's Name] as her very good friend ... could have a word with her and offer her a few ideas that could make a real difference to her frame of mind? ... Could you suggest some alternatives to 'What if it all goes wrong?' and 'What if I can't manage it?' [Pause] I wonder whether it would be better to suggest 'What if some things turn out better than expected?' or even 'What if everything turns out reasonably well?' ... Well, you are her wise friend and advisor who knows her best so why don't you decide? Take as long as you like and let me know once you've offered her some really useful 'What ifs'. [Pause]

That's fine .... Now, how about floating up above her ... and then floating down behind her and taking a moment or two to get a different angle on things from this perspective. ... Can you become aware of the unhelpful thinking patterns that have been used in the past so that [Client's Name] can *avoid these in the future* and *allow some of the positive 'what ifs' to occur more easily* ... when you notice those negative patterns now it might even strike you as odd that [Client's Name] didn't see them before but the important thing is that ... from now on ... with your help ... she can do her best to *avoid them and try out new patterns that are more appropriate* at this time in her life. So take a moment or two just to observe ... and to listen to old thoughts ... to *become aware of old automatic yet outdated responses* so that ... in a moment ... you can pass on your observations. Nod your head when you have become aware of them. [Pause]

These questions can either be considered silently or be answered out loud as the patient prefers. Allow plenty of pauses for thought

Negative 'what if' thinking is very common in depressed patients. Incorporate 'what ifs' **into a more positive framework rather than suggest stopping them all together**

Encouragement to change expectations

'Behind' will often indicate time in the past. If your consulting room/office allows, you can walk around so that your voice comes from the suggested direction, which enhances the effect

Avoid unhelpful patterns and try out new ones. Discuss these beforehand

So, having found some old unhelpful thinking patterns and some ineffective responses I wonder if you can point them out to [Client's Name] and see if, between you, you can come up with an alternative or two to try out over the next few days/week(s) which will help *lift her spirits and perhaps get her involved in something a bit more active* … take all the time you need and let me know when you are ready to move on. [Pause]

Embedded commands
Activity is helpful

Thank you. Well done. So now it's time for you to float up again … bringing all your interesting insights with you … and just before we finish today … float out into the future now and see what it's like now that [Client's Name] has listened to your thoughts and advice and is more aware of her inner strength … using some positive 'what ifs' … and generally looking at things with more optimism and positivity … notice some of the differences that she has made to her daily life … are there a few smiles? … Does she seem to be more outwardly focused? … What do you think other people are noticing about her?

'just before we finish' **alerts the patient to the imminent ending of the session and concentrates the mind and, possibly, increases receptivity to suggestion**

Well, it really is time now for you, Observant Part, to float back from the future into the present time. Float right back down inside [Client's Name] … bringing all those insights and those useful pieces of learning with you … store them in a special place inside where you can *make use of them everyday* … to *lift your spirits* and help you *feel more able to cope* … help you *feel more able to deal with things resourcefully* even if things don't go quite according to plan … and of course … now that your plan is 'that you can deal with things even when they don't go according to plan' … you realize that … coping positively when things don't go to plan, actually *is* your plan … so you will find that unexpected things are going according to plan and you can *deal with them very well indeed.*

Reintegration of parts

Embedded suggestion to deal with setbacks resourcefully

This wording is intentionally confusing in order to increase the likelihood that the final suggestion, 'deal with them very well indeed' **will be accepted**

Take a moment or two now to see how you can put some of these strategies into practice in some very real specific occasions in your life that will be occurring in the next week/couple of weeks ... what difference is this making to you ... to your children/husband/partner/colleagues? ... How is your voice? ... How are they reacting? ... How are you responding to a setback now you feel more resourceful? ... Mmm ... interesting.

Mention very specific useful pre-elicited situations and actions. Or, afterwards, enquire what occasions she was imagining to further reinforce their occurrence

Presupposition

So just as soon as your unconscious mind has assimilated all of this ... your conscious mind will begin to notice that you feel the energy returning to your limbs ... *your whole body and mind ... all parts of you working well together as one complete, integrated whole* and back here in the present in the room with me. Your eyes will want to reopen and see the world around you from a more balanced and optimistic point of view.

Further reintegration of parts

Go to a more formal trance reorientation if appropriate

Jigsaw

This script uses the metaphor of starting to piece together a jigsaw (of life) and rearranging or replacing individual pieces. It has both visual and kinaesthetic appeal.

This may be the time for you to rest for a while … relax a little and give yourself a break from those sad/uncomfortable/overwhelming/depressing/heavy feelings that you were telling me about … just a few minutes where you can *take some time out for a little comfort* … as you *make yourself more comfortable* right now … *settle yourself down* … noticing where the very first comfortable feelings begin … *observing the comfort developing as it spreads out* … perhaps like a ripple in a pond … so that every place that it touches in *your mind and body is soothed and warmed* … just a little time for relaxing and calming the body … just a little time for relaxing and calming the mind … just a little time for you to *enjoy the rest* … and while you're resting you can allow yourself a pleasant daydream … of something that pleases you … some special place that pleases you … perhaps where you can stroll … or sit … or lie down … or even float … as you allow your mind to ponder on the words that you hear … absorb the ideas that are right for you … integrate them into your own way of thinking … just resting and relaxing and maybe beginning to *enjoy this daydream* for a while.

And … as you daydream … I wonder if you … like me … can remember doing a jigsaw … (or can just imagine doing a jigsaw) … and how overwhelming it can feel at first when you look at all those pieces and … possibly even doubt that they can all fit together … but … then you pick up a few pieces here and there and parts of the picture begin to *make a little more sense* … and of course each of us has our preferred ways to *make a start* … piece together the edges … keep checking back to see that they fit in with the bigger picture … or possibly start with the main theme … and *sort out all those bits first* …

Paces the feelings they have described

Suggestions for comfort (physical and emotional) are normally well accepted by people who are depressed

Note the ambiguity of 'enjoy the rest' **(relaxation)/**'enjoy the rest' **(of the session)**

Embedded commands encourage taking action … it doesn't actually matter where they start

of course the important thing is to *make a start ... start anywhere at all that feels easiest to you ...* and when you find that larger/*whole sections are beginning to come together ...* how *immensely satisfying that can be.*

And, although you might think it could be a bit of a cliché ... but often life *is* a bit of a cliché ... I find that looking at life/a situation as if it were a jigsaw can be quite therapeutic ... so how about looking at *your situation* now just like a jigsaw picture ... a rather different kind of jigsaw where you can take out certain pieces and choose from alternative pieces that seem to be more appropriate. ... Now it's true that some of those parts cannot easily be changed because they are under the control of someone or something else, but ... (isn't it interesting?) ... now you *stop* and *really* look at things from this *new perspective* ... how you can see that there *are* things that *can* be changed ... little things here and there that can *start a chain reaction* ... just as merely moving *one* domino can *create a totally different scenario* ... sometimes a seemingly small shift in thinking can *create a massive shift* in our ability to *cope with something or cope with someone in a far more resourceful way* ... a way which is more hopeful ... or more light hearted ... or more resilient ... or allows us to *feel more protected* ... or *feel more in control* ... or *feel more at ease* ... or *feel that we have the inner resources to come through this time stronger and wiser.*

Look at the different pieces to select from ... they're all about you ... there are ones where you *look more confident* ... ones where *you are feeling more resourceful* ... ones where somehow *you have become more assertive* ... ones where *you have become more optimistic* ... ones where you have *cast aside any possible 'victim thinking'* and decide to *take some action* ... ones where you are able to *be so much more resilient* ... so things which used to worry/scare/depress you seem to have so much

> **Pre-empts and 'depotentiates' the idea of a cliché**

> 'stop' **can interrupt the thinking pattern.**
> 'and *really* look at things' **suggests that they weren't really looking closely before**

> **Use your voice to emphasize all the embedded commands**

less impact now. … Take an even closer look and find any unhelpful pieces which you can *replace with a more positive attitude … a more resourceful outlook* … where you think laterally/outside the box and see more possibilities to *take some positive action.* … Just have a look around and try some of the pieces out for size … how do they feel? … And notice the different effect they have not only on you but on others around you too … take all the time you need to rearrange all the pieces so that they work best for you and then stand back and view the larger picture … noticing the changes and *how satisfying they can be*. [Pause] And when you're ready … walk forward and take a step into the scene as it now is … *be there now* … aware of more resources … take a walk around … how does it feel? … Notice how well all these new pieces work for you and be proud of yourself for having fitted them into your life so well … listen to your inner voice … stronger … more hopeful … observing opportunities. [Pause]

Visual

Kinaesthetic

Auditory

And do know that you can revisit this jigsaw in your mind whenever you want to … reinforcing what you like and what is good … changing and improving anything that you want to. But for now … it's nearly time to reorient to the room so take just a few moments more to allow a little more light into this place … so that *things do look brighter* … so as you *bring these feelings back to the room with you* … maybe wanting to stretch and wriggle your fingers and your toes … you can *become aware that your spirits have been lifting* and will *continue to lift a little more each day* as your unconscious mind lives out and adapts as necessary this more resourceful jigsaw of your mind … and your eyes can *open just* as soon as you *feel this sense of renewed hope* and energy within.

Encourages independence and ongoing ability to change

Immediate post-hypnotic suggestion

Go to a more formal trance reorientation if appropriate

Mental movie

The listener is encouraged to be the writer, director and lead actor in a movie of a more satisfying way of life.

And as you are just relaxing comfortably there with your eyes comfortably closed ... I want to talk to you about the reason that you have chosen to be here with me today ... I believe you are tired of living with that cloud hanging over you and you want to *be free of those miserable thoughts* that were dragging you down and you want to be rid of the feeling that you had no control over them. ... you *have come to a realisation* that now is the time you want to *lift your mood* ... time to *find some more active enjoyment in your world* ... *enjoy some of the things* ... *enjoy some of the people* ... *around you* ... *find pleasure in some of the everyday aspects of your life* as well as in the more special ones.

> Reminds them of their aim and that they made a deliberate choice to come for treatment
>
> You are 'pacing' their depressed feelings first so they feel understood
>
> Acknowledges the decision to change is their own and then embeds suggestions which should have general appeal

And one of the interesting things about listening in this pleasant, daydreamy, relaxing state is that your unconscious mind has been becoming more and more wonderfully creative and receptive to positive ideas and suggestions ... which can *improve your life visibly and tangibly.* ... Your ability to *see things from a different perspective* allows you *get a new slant on things* ... *get things into proportion* and *talk to yourself in a far more supportive way.*

> Very unthreatening state
>
> Seeds the idea of increasing creativity and receptivity of the unconscious mind, which will be developed further VAK expressions give more appeal

And here's the time to use that enhanced creativity of yours ... you can be the writer, the director and ... even enjoy being the lead actor in your very own mental movie ... Take a moment now to *consider consciously* those things you would like to change about how you think ... about how you feel ... change how you see things to help you *enjoy your life more* ... Remember that this is about how *you* would prefer to feel and to think positively ... *not* how you can change other people's behaviour.

> Validates the use of the conscious mind in the trance state (some people persist in believing the myth of complete unconsciousness in the hypnotic state)
>
> Reminder that we can only change ourselves, not other people

Take another moment now to reassure *your uncon-scious* mind, which is always listening, that you *do indeed want to create that change* where you can *allow some positivity into your life.* Just assume that your unconscious mind is listening … and mentally and silently explain in your own words that you want to *let go of depressing thoughts and feelings* and *take on more hopeful, assured thoughts* in their place. [Pause]

Participation now of the unconscious mind

And now is the time to create and direct your movie. … Have yourself, the actor … use a new strategy to *raise your spirits* in everyday situations in your life … that will help you to *notice some good things around you … actively seek out and focus on more positive aspects in your life … find a way to rise above those things that used to get you down … and take them in your stride.* You are the director of the film so this is your opportunity to coach the actor how to play the part convincingly … so that every gesture, every facial expression, all the body language reflects the inner positivity. Run the mental movie through of an average day including lots of detail and check that the tone of voice as well as the words sound positive and optimistic and check the body language too. [Pause]

Embedded commands

You may keep these suggestions general or use pre-elicited information to guide them through the process, e.g. see yourself getting up in the morning with more energy feeling lighter and brighter, moving more quickly … find it seems perfectly natural to pick up that phone and suggest a meeting … sense the impetus to get started on the washing/ the new sales strategy/ gardening/writing etc

Rerun it and rerun it … getting the actor to improve it every time until you are completely satisfied with the performance. [Pause]

Repetition reinforces acceptance but this time refrain from any guidance. Allow plenty of time for them to do this

Great … so now you have used your conscious mind to direct exactly *what* you want to happen … *how* you want it to happen … and … (as this is so important to you) … just give a quick reminder now to your unconscious that this **is** what *you really, truly want* … so now you can trust it to work out a whole new strategy to *raise you up* … to *create a brighter future* … just remind it now. [Pause] That's it … and with this new strategy you will find that you *take things more lightly* … as though a weight has been

You are getting them to invest personally in these decisions

lifting so much more easily from your shoulders than ever you thought it could … couldn't it? So, from now on … you will be aware of a greater sense of hopefulness … you will become aware of a spark of positive energy glowing inside you … which encourages you to *be more outwardly focused* every day … you will experience feelings of increased confidence and control … which will enable you to *enjoy* being *yourself so much more than before* … you will stay more confident and at ease … no matter where you are … no matter when you are there … no matter who you're with … no matter when you are alone … you will be feeling positive inside.

Ego strengthening

And while you're asleep each night your mind will be strengthening your strategy … strengthening you at the inner … unconscious level … without your even knowing *how* at the conscious level … it will just happen while you breathe naturally … breathe out any possible despondent feelings … breathe in a sense of optimism so that every day … all day … you will have increased feelings of positivity and confidence … resilience too … which will enable you to *feel more on top of things* than before … because the fact is that you can *cope better with any situation* when *you are lighter and brighter* … *you find you can cope far more easily with any situation* you find yourself in during your daily life.

Strengthening of unconscious resources

So just before we finish I would like you to float forward a little way into your brighter future and when you are there … now … look around and see for yourself those things in your mental film that have actually materialised … get a sense of yourself and notice *how you are indeed feeling more resilient inside* … perhaps even taking a pride in your ability to make those changes even though it took a certain effort on your part. Does it surprise you to notice yourself handling tricky situations far more optimistically and confidently than you would have imagined back then? Look at your face … how much more animated it has become … more open … more

Either include some pre-elicited desired activities and behaviours or simply allow them to fill in the details in their own mind

VAK gives extra appeal

smiling even … notice how all of your body seems so much more at ease and yet has an energy there too … listen to your voice with that note of strength and vitality in it … and of course … now you are sleeping so much better, it's perfectly natural that you wake up feeling rested with a greater sense of energy and optimism as you look forward to the day ahead.

Presupposition of better sleep

The really important thing to be fully aware of is … that the more often you use your conscious mind to direct your positive future … the more you will be able to trust your inner mind to *carry out your wishes* and help you *create your own brighter future. The more often you practise thinking optimistically with your conscious mind … the more optimistic you will become deep inside,* and the more you will find you are increasingly able to cope with any situation you face in your everyday life … cope with anybody … cope with anything so much more confidently than ever you thought you could … and just as soon as your unconscious mind and your conscious mind have found the way to work in harmony to *ensure all of this happens* … you will *begin to notice the energy now beginning to spread around your body* … your fingers perhaps beginning to notice it first … then your hands and arms wanting to stretch … and your eyelids wanting to open as you become aware of the spark of optimism growing inside that feels really good … and when you reorient to the room with me you will feel completely refreshed and alert.

Reminder to practise at the conscious level

The benefits of practice

Go to a more formal trance reorientation if appropriate

Sleep

Face anxieties in the daytime and relax the mind at night

This script is suitable for people whose minds go over and over anxieties and problems which surface at night time thus preventing them from sleeping. It gives a strategy for letting go of night time worries and concerns and also gives positive suggestions for relaxation and sleep

Perhaps now is the time for you take a moment to think about how you have been consciously fighting with your unconscious mind ... your unconscious mind has been trying to help you by reminding you that there are matters of importance that it believes you need to address ... so why not ... *stop now* ... and consider for a moment or two how helpful ... or indeed unhelpful ... is your current strategy of refusing to face up to these problems in the daytime. [Pause] Now that you *really think about it* ... have you discovered yet that this strategy actually doesn't work very well for you? [You will almost certainly get a 'Yes' answer.]

'stop now' **is a pattern interrupt**

Reframes sleeping difficulties as a strategy of refusing to face problems in the daytime. 'Changing a strategy' may likely be better accepted than 'overcoming a sleeping problem'

So, you agree that a different strategy would work better for you ... that's good ... now first I want to reassure you that there are many different ways of using the hypnotic state to help *deal with anxieties and help with solving problems* and perhaps later ... or at another time of your choosing ... we can look at some of your particular worries together ... but there are also ways to *feel more comfortable at night while* you *wait* for problems to be worked out ... so why don't we look at those right now?

Embedded command to 'deal with anxieties', but also to '*feel more comfortable at night*' while waiting for this to happen

And I'm sure you'd agree that ... as you have been so short of sleep ... this may well be the time for you to let yourself find a way to rest ... right now and enjoy some comfortable relaxation as you absorb this simple ... yet tried and tested strategy ... no

The suggestion to rest should be well accepted

'tried and tested' **sounds very reassuring**

66

need to try too hard to concentrate on the words … merely let the voice itself relax you deeper and deeper and … as you do go deeper and deeper now with each out breath … I wonder if you are noticing yourself following every word and absorbing the strategy into your inner store of automatic strategies/ habits … or whether you are simply enjoying the relaxing … knowing that there is no need to concern yourself with this consciously … as all the absorbing will happen at the unconscious level.

Double bind; the strategy can be absorbed consciously or unconsciously

Every night as you go to bed, the very important thing to do is to make an appointment with yourself for the following day … where you will sit down and give your full attention to any concerns that previously you had been avoiding … set yourself a specific time which you will keep to, come what may … so have a notepad by your bed and if any stray thought should disturb you in any way, simply write down the key words and phrases of those conscious worries or concerns … however trivial they might seem … so that your unconscious mind can relax … because … in this way it will know these points are recorded and then it will relax as it has no need to keep reminding your conscious mind of them … and as your mind relaxes more and more automatically as you go to bed you will find that your body … indeed your whole system … enjoys this time of comfort and ease … comfort and ease gently developing as you rest so naturally there.

This can also be discussed and clarified pre- or post-trance

This is why it is so important to set yourself a specific time for the following day when you will sit down and take out the notepad and carefully consider the points that you have written on it, and give them your full attention … at a time when you're refreshed and ready to deal with them … feeling stronger and thinking more clearly after a good night's sleep … that way, you see things more clearly, and get them into proportion. It's very important that you do take the time and trouble to do this at the exact time you decided … because … only in this way will your

Presupposition of a good night's sleep

VK

unconscious mind know it can trust your conscious mind ... and your conscious mind can trust your unconscious to let you *sleep in a very calm and easy way*.

Now I'm not going to suggest that you *sleep immediately as you settle/snuggle down in your bed* ... since everyone needs a little time to wind down and relax ... only that you take some time to enjoy the comfort ... as you ... calmly and patiently ... allow sleep to come upon you ... and as you become increasingly aware of the comfort spreading calm, that ever growing feeling of calm comfort allows you to fully enjoy the relaxation all the way through ... whether you're in the stage of drifting ... or dreaming ... or sleeping deeply ... or sleeping lightly ... or dreaming again ... or drifting again so comfortably ... so calmly ... we all drift through the stages of sleep ... drifting down ... drifting up ... drifting down again and drifting away ... deeper and deeper ... of course, if there were any genuine need ... you would, naturally, wake ... but normally you can stay quietly calm and comfortable all night through ... quietly calm in your body ... quietly calm in your mind ... and even though you are asleep ... a part of you can be aware you are sleeping ... strange how you can be aware you are sleeping or is it that you are dreaming you're sleeping? But what a nice dream ... and ... if you should rouse for a moment or two ... you will hear my words ... 'quietly ... calm' ... and they will seem to come from the very core of you ... and whether or not you experience them as my words or your own internal words ... you will turn over and drift back to sleep ... quietly calm all night through.

And now you are using your new strategy of facing up to concerns and dealing with things in the daytime, the quality of your *sleep will improve every night* ... and as the quality of *your sleep improves*, so the quality of your everyday life improves ... you will *feel refreshed when you wake* after a good

---

Intentional confusion prior to the embedded command for sleep

'Now I'm *not* going to suggest' **uses the negative to discharge any possible resistance. The embedded command** *'sleep immediately'* *follows straight on*

'allow sleep to come upon you' **suggests all that needs to be done is to give permission for it to happen rather than its being a struggle**

People often report that they don't sleep at all whereas, in truth, they are napping and waking. This gives suggestions for being more aware of sleep

Reinforcement of strategy

night's sleep … with a feeling that you can *cope with things more easily than before* … you will *feel more energised and in control in your daily life* … you will *see things clearly* … you will *think in a more positive way* … you will *get on with things that need to be done* and get a feeling of satisfaction as you complete them … and now that *you are sleeping so much better,* you find that you have an altogether more positive outlook in so many ways.

Ego strengthening

Note the presupposition
'now that *you are sleeping so much better*'

Soon we will be drawing the session to a close … so you may like to spend a few moments/minutes now seeing in your mind's eye a dream-like sequence of everything we've talked about … images, thoughts, realisations … happening gently … with you relaxing gently in the evening … a sense of calm and contentment at night … night-time becomes calm time … calm and comfortable time … no time at all before you drift off into a dream. [Pause]

Pause for reflection

Go to a suitable trance reorientation

Practical ways to improve the quality of sleep

This script gives direct suggestions for promoting good quality sleep and also links normal bedtime routines to relaxation and drowsiness.

And feeling comfortably, pleasantly relaxed and at ease now ... you may be surprised when you hear me say that I'm *not* going to tell you that *every night when you go to bed you will fall asleep within minutes* ... but I *am* going to say that *every night it will seem increasingly natural that you can feel relaxed and calm and at ease* ... as indeed you are now ... and because *you will feel so relaxed and so calm and at ease* ... the exact moment when you fall asleep will no longer seem so important ... *you will just be enjoying the sense of peaceful relaxation and inner comfort* ... *each night you will enjoy this state of rest and relaxation a little bit more* ... *and a little bit more* ... also knowing that you are putting steps in place to *improve the quality of your sleep* ... so you can *really relax* as you *drift and dream* ... *patiently waiting for sleep to come upon you* ... *thinking to yourself that you are really enjoying the relaxation and the comfort.*

'I'm *not* going to tell you ...' **confounds their expectations and more easily allows the following embedded command to bypass their conscious awareness**

This places the emphasis on rest, calm and comfort rather than on sleep itself

And there are many straightforward ways to *improve the quality of your sleep* ... some you know and some you may be hearing for the first time ... and some you may have known but forgotten you have known ... and now ... you will not only know ... but also *implement each little detail* and so ensure the quality of your *sleep will improve every night* ... and as the quality of *your sleep improves*, so the quality of your everyday life improves ... you will *feel refreshed when you wake* after a good night's sleep ... with a feeling that you're going to *enjoy your day* ... you will *feel more energised in your daily life* ... you will *see things clearly* ... you will *think in a positive way* ... you will *get on with things that need to be done* and get a feeling of satisfaction as you complete them ... now *you are sleeping so much*

You maintain rapport by acknowledging that they will possibly already know some of these things

This section contains lots of embedded commands and it also presents a positive outcome to look forward to right at the start of the session

Presupposition of sleep

better … you find that you have an altogether more positive outlook in so many ways.

And we all know that in the hypnotic state we can *relax in a calm and comfortable way* … but did you also know that it is a state where you can *focus and absorb ideas* with or without the need for conscious concentration? … Your unconscious mind becomes more attentive while your conscious mind can *drift and dream* … so it's nice to know that you can *let your conscious mind drift down to some calm place in you* while your unconscious mind can *focus and absorb every word* as you relax … and drift down … drift up … drift away.

And as you drift and relax a little deeper now, I'll remind you of some of the things I am sure you already know … how in the evening it's so much better to spend the last couple of hours enjoying relaxing, physically and mentally, so as not to over-stimulate your mind … preparing yourself for the comfortable rest and calm ahead … so when you read or watch television, choose content which is relaxing and not mentally stimulating before bed … exercise should be taken ideally in the late afternoon or very early evening and preferably in the fresh air … avoid mid to late evening exercise in order to give time for your body to reduce its temperature and so encourage better sleep.

Each day you will be finding that it is becoming natural and automatic to choose drinks which are free from caffeine in the evening and, certainly, avoid or go easy on alcohol since it stimulates the bladder and the heartbeat too … and you certainly wouldn't want to be aroused after you've been able to gently doze off into a very comfortable state of relaxation.

A generalisation that most people would accept

This may possibly be a new idea which also takes the pressure off 'having' to relax. They can 'focus' rather than relax if they prefer

'Reminding' is often more acceptable than 'telling'

This section can also be personalised according to pre-elicited information

Apparently a lower core temperature is associated with the onset of sleep

This section can also be personalised according to pre-elicited information

Presupposition of the ability to 'gently doze off'

Because your mind and your body work in harmony ... of course your thoughts are affected by your physical feelings ... and naturally your physical feelings are affected by your thoughts ... so you can make a decision to *keep your bedroom calm and peaceful so that your mind associates your bedroom with sleep* ... and *your body associates your bedroom with sleep* ... so you can *make the decision* to keep television, computers and even books in rooms which you associate with wakefulness ... and increasingly *your mind associates your bedroom as* ... yes ... *a soothing haven of peace that promotes easy, restful sleep.*

One generalisation is followed by another and linked to another until eventually the suggestion to remove mentally stimulating TV, computers etc. from the bedroom is made. Hopefully this makes it more easily accepted

You will have discussed the advisability of this in your pre-trance discussion

In fact, now that *your mind understands that your bedroom is the place for easy, restful sleep* ... and your body naturally follows your thought ... as soon as you open the door to your bedroom, you will *notice a feeling of pleasant calm coming over you* ... and when it's time for bed ... this association becomes even stronger ... so as soon as you open the door at bedtime, *an urge to yawn will come over you* ... and you know what a yawn is like ... the harder you try to control it ... *the stronger the impulse to yawn becomes* ... and that rather pleasant feeling of drowsiness seems to be spreading through your entire system ... each step of your bedtime routine seems to be a further trigger for feelings of calm and drowsiness ... now I am *not* saying that ... because you *feel so drowsy,* you will skip certain aspects of that routine ... only that you will likely *feel the temptation because the feelings of drowsiness are so insistent* ... but you will resist the temptation to skip over them, hard though that may be ... and ... as you clean your teeth for example, you will certainly be feeling glad that you won't have to wait much longer for the delight of that happy, comfy, relaxing feeling as you slip under the covers ... and when your face touches the pillow, it will be such a welcome relief as you *welcome that wonderful peaceful feeling of being in bed.* Just being there in this peaceful, calm place is so relaxing ... you *feel*

This section links drowsiness to normal bedtime routines

The law of reversed effect

so at ease in your surroundings wherever you are … just getting into bed and laying your head on the pillow … nothing bothers you now … nothing disturbs this wonderful sense of inner peace and calm … you really enjoy being in bed.

Merely being in bed can be relaxing. Takes the pressure off needing to sleep

Over the forthcoming days and weeks you will become aware that your expectations are in a process of change … in fact your expectations are changing in many ways … you *expect to feel more positive* and so you *do feel more positive* … you expect to *feel more refreshed in the morning* and so *you do feel more refreshed in the morning* … and cope more easily with thoughts that need your focus and attention … and when you go to bed at night *you expect to sleep well* and so you *do sleep well* and … because you *expect to sleep well* … and you *do sleep well* … you will find that *your mind can drift onto things that are far more relaxing to dream about* and I'm wondering how soon it will be before *all these things have become a normal and natural part of what happens* and you just do them automatically without even thinking about them at all.

Soon we will be drawing the session to a close … so you may like to spend a few moments now seeing in your mind's eye any changes you will make to your bedroom to make it more peaceful … bringing a sense of calm and contentment as soon as you open the door at bedtime … night-time becomes calm time … calm and comfortable time … no time at all before you drift off into a dream. [Pause]

Go to a suitable trance reorientation

Absorb the knowledge of sleep

Drift down to that place in you where you can expand the horizons of your mind ... and just have a look at the horizon now ... and notice the gentle fading light there as the sun is going down ... this gentle fading light contains the secrets of sleep ... every night the sun goes down and signals the beginnings of sleep ... people all around respond to the signal of fading light ... and ... as you see that light over there, you are beginning to feel drawn towards it ... floating over to it ... somehow knowing that it holds everything you need to know ... of quiet and calm ... everything you need to feel of calm and comfort ... and of course you don't need to know this consciously ... simply allow your unconscious to have that experience of sleep so that it can experience ... and re-experience time after time ... these wonderful feelings every time you choose to sleep ... so you can now gently step into that dim light ... or float into it ... or dream your way into it ... that's it ... feeling it ... gently touching your skin ... with sleep ... understanding at last at a deep inner level the full knowledge of sleep ... absorbing the skills of sleep and welcoming in the wonderful habit of rest and sleep for the rest of your life so that your unconscious allows your body and your mind to *respond spontaneously to signals for sleep whenever and wherever it's safe for you to do so* ... without any conscious effort at all ... so that ... from now on ... when it's the right time and right place for you to sleep ... you will find that you can sleep anywhere, sleep any place you want when it's safe for you to do so ... your mind will relax spontaneously ... your body will relax spontaneously when it's the right time ... so you are in time ... to let every single muscle and nerve of your body relax and let go of any stored tension or stress of the day ... you can't actually avoid it ... when it's your chosen time to sleep ... it just happens ... your mind and body respond automatically ... the harder you were even to try to resist ... the more that sense of drifty, dreamy, drowsy sleepiness

Presupposition that the 'place in you where you can *expand the horizons of your mind'* **exists**

Sleep anywhere they want

The law of reversed effect

74

will come upon you … and you will just give in to the pleasant feeling and drift off to sleep quietly and calmly … sleep quietly and calmly all night through … stay quietly calm … and if you should rouse for a moment you will hear my voice reminding you that you can sleep anywhere … sleep any place … sleep any time you like … so you do … turn over and drift back down again to enjoy a wonderful deep sleep.

'give in' **suggests that sleep is difficult to resist**

Avoids suggestions too specifically linked to the client's own bedroom

And as you are sleeping easily and comfortably each night … it's good to know that your unconscious mind is exploring every aspect of sleep … discovering new ways for you to *relax even deeper and let go of unwanted* tensions … let go of unwanted thoughts in the evening … *deal with any concerns in the daytime* so you can *rest comfortably, calmly and tranquilly all night through.*

Presupposition of sleep

The unconscious mind is continuing to find ways for deeper relaxation and release of tension

I invite you now to *create … consciously … some kind of sense or picture of yourself,* lying there … at bedtime … enjoying the comfort … some people can *see themselves*, just loving the calm, inner tranquillity … other people just *feel it on the inside* … other people seem to *hear a whisper of inner calm* … whatever you experience … *it seems so good to be in this place* … luxuriating in the feelings of rest and calm … any thoughts seeming to drift off with your breathing … more and more pleasantly aware of how comfortable … how comforting it is to be here … drifting up … drifting down … drifting back up again … drifting away … drifting off … until the next thing you are aware of is that it's morning and *you wake feeling refreshed and revitalised after a good night's sleep* … full of energy, feeling full of calm confidence … ready to enjoy your day … knowing that you've had a wonderful night's rest … and each day you become more and more calm and confident … that each night … you become more and more able to drift off … into a wonderful, quietly calm sleep.

Future pacing

VAK enriches the experience

Encourages the natural process of the mind drifting as sleep approaches

Now, of course, I don't know ... and I don't need to *know exactly* at which point *you will realise that all those old bedtime concerns are a thing of the past* ... whether it was immediately or after a few days or weeks that you were able to just *forget all about them/that period in your life* in the delight of feeling so comfortable now ... so confident ... so calm and at ease ... day ... evening ... night ... now you have absorbed the full knowledge of sleep at the unconscious level ... you will feel pleasantly comfortable ... confident ... calm and at ease ... a little more each day ... a little more each night ... not only at a deep inner level but at the outer level too.

'a little more each day ... a little more each night' **takes away the pressure to see immediate results**

Go to a suitable trance reorientation

Sexual Issues

Considerations

Reduced sexual performance can occur as a result of a physical, psychological or emotional problem such as diabetes or depression. Anti-hypertensive medication or anti-androgen medication in the case of prostate cancer will also have an effect, as indeed can smoking. Therefore it is suggested that the client seeks a referral from their medical practitioner before undergoing hypnotherapy treatment.

Generally speaking it is advisable to undertake specific training before treating patients with long-standing sexual dysfunction.

Inevitably in a general collection of this kind, these scripts cannot be 'in depth' but they may be found useful where problems may arise from a degree of performance anxiety and a temporary lack of confidence arising from mild stress or overtiredness or minor ill health. The scripts are intended as part rather than the whole of a treatment.

People vary greatly in their hypnotic response and in their receptivity to different approaches. Some clients will respond very well to ego strengthening, positive suggestion, metaphor and visualisation; others respond to cognitive behaviour therapy whereas others may be better helped by approaches that seek out originating events and help to heal old emotional wounds.

Lessen the effect of negative mental images in erectile dysfunction is helpful where the client is beset by mental images and negative thoughts of failure, both past and projected future failures.

The deceptively simple technique of progression into the future adopted in the script *Problem resolved* can be quite powerful since it implants the idea that the problem has long since been resolved and it allows you to look back from a far more empowered perspective than a problem-laden one. It can be adapted for use with different sexual issues.

Hypnotic dreams is a metaphorical extract intended to increase arousal, primarily in women. Additional metaphors have been added which are perhaps more suitable for men and also for ejaculatory inhibition.

Lessen the effect of negative mental images in erectile dysfunction

This script deals with eliminating or reducing the negative effect of mental pictures and unhelpful self-talk associated with past and/ or prospective failure, both of which are usually present in sexual performance anxiety. It is useful to elicit these in the pre-trance discussion so that the client can more easily follow the instructions in the script.

And feeling pleasantly aware of the beginnings of a somewhat altered state of awareness ... *noticing* ... as we go along ... that your ability to *see things from a different perspective* becomes enhanced ... you may also like to notice how you *discover access to unconscious strengths and resources* ... understand, for example, how you can use your mind's very natural ability to *make mental pictures to direct your body* ... sometimes people do this unintentionally and negatively but ... in the powerful state of hypnosis ... you can *do this positively today ... and everyday* ... and so *achieve the excellent results you desire*.

> A 'beginning' **implies there will be a continuation of the process**

Consider for a moment how some people worry about something stressful ... and then they develop a very physical response of a headache or acid indigestion for example ... a very direct (although negative) mind-body reaction ... whereas, on a more positive note ... people can *physically feel as though a weight has been lifted from them* when they suddenly *see there is a completely different solution to a problem* ... one of the processes going on at the unconscious level is that we see mental images ... we have thoughts that *pop up* all the time ... we talk to ourselves ... and these pictures and this self-talk directly affect the way our bodies respond so we need to *organise these pictures and thoughts with a bit of simple and direct training* ... (or retraining) ... to ensure that they *do a good job* ... *easily get the result you want* and the wonderful thing is ...

> **Scattered throughout the text are words or phrases encouraging arousal**

that this heightened state of hypnotic awareness ...
makes it easier to get the result you want.

So let's consider what *you can change today* ...
how about substituting mental pictures of what you
actually want in place of images that you don't want
... I imagine *it must be a great relief* to know that
in the hypnotic state *you can change those mental
pictures ... you can change that way of thinking*
... in a way that will *give you an altogether more
confident and enjoyable sexual experience ...* you'll
find yourself easily more able to *enjoy getting and
maintaining an erection hardly even thinking about it*
... and what once seemed difficult will now *feel hard
yet easy at the same time ... increasingly easily hard
(every time).*

Introducing the idea of *relief* that this can all be changed in the hypnotic state

And I think you're going to enjoy being surprised by
the ease with which you can *reorganise and rewire
your thoughts* in this special state of enhanced hypnotic thinking ... just following the simple conscious
instructions and allowing *your unconscious* to *create
an automatic process* which *will have a gratifying
effect on your performance* in the most delightful
of ways ... so first things first ... allow yourself just
for a moment or two ... (really, it will be just for a
moment or two) ... to *get up* that unwanted picture
in your mind that you told me about ... tell me when
you have it ... alright ... now bear with this for a
few moments while we get all the information you
need to *change this mental image* ... hear again any
negative thoughts, blaming self-talk and unhelpful
self-doubt and feelings in the body that had accompanied the image ... let yourself be aware of them
too and tell me when you recognize them ... OK ...
so this is what we do ... this is how to *change all
that.*

Visual

Auditory

Kinaesthetic

Look at that negative mental picture and imagine filling it with light ... a light which is so light and bright
... let it get so light that *the picture begins to disintegrate* so that as you look at it you can no longer see

Visual

the image … (a bit like looking into the sun) … and, now I'd like you to let this same white light fill your ears and blur out … fade out … any trace of thought … your ears are filled with a white light that in this very unusual way cuts through the thought and causes it to disintegrate …and what's more … this amazing white light *can sear through any uncertainty anywhere in the body … feel it zapping that doubt-ful feeling even now* … good … let more and more bright white light in … so that *the whole picture, the negative thoughts and the feelings disappear* … tell me when you can no longer see the image … that's right … *you can no longer see the image* … so you see nothing at all … well done … now try to find the original image again … and … if you can … as soon as you see it … even if it's already a bit blurred … begin to fill the image with light until *it completely obliterates the picture … obliterates the thoughts and obliterates the negative feelings* … and tell me when you've done it.

Auditory

Kinaesthetic

This process will be repeated several times. If the client says the image is still there, explain it will lessen as you continue

'try to get the original image' suggests the original image may already have changed. (The eventual aim, of course, is to lose the negative mental trigger image)

Repeat this procedure several times until the client is no longer able to recreate the original image and accompanying thoughts and feelings (or, they are very much weaker than they used to be)

Great … you're doing this so well … just a bit more to add to the process … we're going to *create a positive exciting image* that you can use in your mind to *replace that old one* … you could make it the image of your partner looking admiringly at you perhaps or you could make it any exciting image you like … after all it's your image and you don't have to tell me what it is … And you can also realise that the white light was acting as a positive filter … not only obliterating negative thought … but also actively encouraging positive thoughts in … so add in an exciting thought … and feel that energy inside … the blood coursing through your veins … a hardening sense of strength … aware that the more you look at your partner/see that mental image, the stronger that erection becomes. Add in anything you want to make this image more exciting and pleasurable to you … that's it … this is the new image … with

Best to use an image suggested by the client

its accompanying thoughts and feelings … that you can store in your mind to trigger the desired response in your body.

Now the final part of the jigsaw … I'd like you once again to try to get up a 'reminder trace' of that old unwanted image in your mind's eye … even though it may be very fragmented indeed … and when you do … fill it with the amazing white light that clears everything out … just as you did before … it clears away pictures … fades away thoughts … zaps doubt and uncertainty … you only see the powerful white light … now look right through the whiteness and you will see the new image … <u>there is your partner looking at you … admiring what they see</u> … this new image ignites an excitement in you … you are aware of a growing sense of arousal … an energy pulsing through your body … the continuing strength of your reaction/erection will now be *effortlessly/pleasingly automatic … no thoughts … only aroused feelings.*

Or, substitute the image your client has selected

It's good to know that the more often you *get up* this mental image … the more you reinforce this trigger of positive performance … and the more you reinforce the trigger … *the more immediate your reaction will become, the stronger your reaction will become and the more long-lasting your erection will become.*

Now just before we finish … I'm going to tell you what top sportsmen in any field do … you might be thinking 'what's that got to do with me?' Well I'll tell you … in addition, of course, to their physical training, sportsmen use their minds to *mentally rehearse how well they intend to perform* … their conscious mind presents the picture to their unconscious minds of exactly how well they will perform … and then it just works automatically because … once their unconscious mind has accepted that picture of peak performance … all the physical body has to do is to *follow on naturally … it happens automatically,*

Presupposition of acceptance

unconsciously and very effectively … it just does it … and … think about it for a moment … these sports-men wouldn't do it if it didn't work and, if *they* can do it … *you can do it* … the golfer can *improve their stroke* … the swimmer can *increase the length of their stroke* … the runner *can improve their staying power* … *there's really no limit on the improvement you can make.*

Apt metaphors

And in the days and the weeks and the months that follow and *you are finding this part of your life more and more satisfying* … I'm wondering whether you will even bother to look back and *congratulate yourself on how well everything has worked out* or whether this will all *seem so natural to you now,* you just *take it in your stride with hardly a thought at all.*

Recommended trance reorientation: *Unconscious continuation*

Problem resolved

Look into the future when the problem has long been resolved.

Although this script contains the occasional example concerning erectile dysfunction, it is not solely intended for this purpose and can be adapted for use with a wide variety of different issues.

Use a suitable induction, generally choosing one with sugges-tions for lightness and lifting rather than for heaviness of limbs if the problem concerns erectile dysfunction. The choice of hand or finger levitation is ideal, if the client is receptive to this approach. This is partly because it is a strong convincer of the power of the mind, partly because it gives an undoubted experience of altered perception in the state of hypnosis and partly because there is an implicit analogy in the lifting and rigidity required both in hand levitation and an erection.

One of the wonderful things about the hypnotic state is that you can *notice yourself drifting in and out of conscious awareness* … sometimes drifting up and sometimes *drifting deeper* … noticing *how pleasant this can feel* as you *experience some of those sen-sations* … and *the alteration of awareness increas-ing* in the most delightful of ways … sometimes you find that *you focus clearly* on every word and other times it seems more that *you are absorbing the most beneficial ideas purely at the unconscious level* … but you can be sure that you will *take up the suggestions in the most effective way for you* and enjoy their *becoming more and more part of your automatic way of responding naturally and easily* … as you enjoy now becoming entranced by the notion that *trance allows so many things* far more easily and effortlessly than conscious trying ever did … allow yourself to <u>fully enjoy the sexual experience</u> <u>and allow your unconscious to maintain that erec-</u><u>tion/let orgasm happen spontaneously without your</u> <u>consciously having to think about it all</u> …

Substitute the client's desired outcome. Stating the goal allows for indirect suggestions to be incorporated even at this initial stage and indicates to the client you have their outcome clearly in mind

I'd like to explain ... or perhaps *remind you* if you already know ... that in the hypnotic state *our powers of creativity are wonderfully enhanced* ... and we *become more aware of our inner strengths and resources* that seem to be more readily available ... or maybe it's just that we *notice they are there* instead of overlooking them in haste ... we also *seem to have an effortless ability to travel back and forth in time in our minds* ... gaining insight and incorporating new learning ... all at the unconscious level that will *show itself in our perceptions ... show itself in our sensations and show itself in our responses* with no conscious effort at all ... and what a relief that can be to *stop consciously trying* to get it right and *allow your unconscious to get it right with no conscious effort on your part at all.*

So while you're relaxing even more comfortably now ... with your breathing, calm and regular ... I'm going to ask your unconscious mind to weave its magic and sift through your thoughts, feelings and memories and just *let any unwanted anxious thoughts, unhelpful tensions or any out-of-date unnecessary fears* be released with your breathing ... carried away and dispersed with the out breath ... while your conscious self is merely aware of a sense of relief as you *drift ... even more deeply ... into the* very special *state* ... and here ... isn't it good to know that your unconscious self can encourage rapid healing of any hurt feelings, disappointments or wounded pride ... *lifting your spirits* and enhancing the process of recovery of energy and enthusiasm ... while your conscious self can just feel grateful that *your unconscious* mind has the wisdom to effect all of this as you *develop more and more pleasurable sensations* ... of trance ... more and more comfortably ... and it's so reassuring ... is it not ... to know *you have all the mental and physical and emotional reserves and resources you need* and I'm now going to ask your unconscious to *delve even deeper* into that wealth of inner strengths and resources to find exactly what you need right now to *ensure that*

Reinforces the concept of the power of both the hypnotic state and the unconscious mind

This seeds the idea of the mental 'ability to travel back and forth in time'

Learning at the unconscious level will show itself at the physical level with no need for conscious effort. This can afford great relief which allows the patient to relax more deeply

Previous conscious attempts to deal with this have probably been unsuccessful so the idea of allowing the unconscious mind to take care of things should come as a relief

those issues are resolved at the innermost level … with every part of you at ease and in agreement with the solution … so that your emotional and physical/ sensual/sexual experience is enhanced in a way *that is deeply satisfying to you* … and you can know that all of this *can happen at the unconscious level* without knowing *how* or *why consciously* … just knowing consciously that your unconscious mind does know how … right now … to *carry out this process so that everything will happen naturally … exactly when and how you want it to* … as you take a few moments now to let it all happen inside … outside your conscious awareness … *enjoying a sense of inner coming together* … understanding that the solution *will emerge effortlessly yet powerfully at the time and place of your choosing.*

And now … I invite you to make use of another amazing ability of your unconscious mind … to *travel forward in time* to a time in the future when … *that issue has long been resolved* … imagine yourself floating forward in time … that's it … floating … float- ing … floating along the line of time … until … you reach the point when that old issue has grown hazy … has become a distant memory almost completely forgotten … it's so long ago … *it's actually hard* to remember quite what it was all about … you are enjoying every aspect of your life fully and completely in the most satisfying of ways now.

This ability was mentioned earlier

Presupposition that the resolution of the problem not only happened but happened long ago

Suggest that the memory has grown 'hazy' **rather than completely forgotten**

And as a natural and normal part of your life now you are enjoying the sexual aspect too … finding it deeply fulfilling … taking a delight in the intimacy … your body understanding instinctively the secrets of arousal … yours … his/her growing arousal. [Pause] Take all the time you want … privately … to enjoy … *really* enjoy … this experience with *every sense* … noticing what you see … noticing what you feel … perhaps even perfumes on the air … perhaps even tasting the delight of success since you learned that special thing of letting the mind relax completely and letting the body take over quite spontaneously.

Offer lots of pauses to encourage full enjoyment of the situation, intensifying the experience by making use of all the senses

Now ... can you please store this experience/'memory from the future' somewhere special inside you so that you *can take it out again and enjoy it whenever you want to* ... maybe even that you could *give others the benefit* of your advice sometime ... who knows? ... And once you are certain that it is safely deep inside ... always to be remembered ... I invite you to *float back along the line of time ... towards but not quite as far as ... the present moment of [today's date]* ... that's it floating ... floating back with wonderful insight and that feeling of satisfaction with how well life turns out ... coming back with that inner and outer certainty ... floating nearly ... but not quite ... all the way back and when you are back as far as you are looking down on the occasion of your very next sexual encounter/experience ... notice how everything is happening just the way you wanted it to be ... *how satisfying this is all the way through ... in every sense ... in every detail ...* and as you look now ... you can understand... *really understand ...* that you *do have the power ... you have the power in you at the unconscious level to let this happen every time you want it to... in just the right way for you ...* that's right. [Pause]

The notion that the client is in the position of being able to give advice to others should be additionally empowering

Looking at the next sexual experience with a clear mental 'future memory of successful outcome' intensifies the effect of this visualisation

So now ... it really is time to float back once again along the line of time all the way back to the present time of [today's date] ... with this knowledge of certainty and confidence deep in your innermost self ... in your mind and in your body ... and good to know that with each and every passing day and night your confidence will increase ... and that confidence encourages you to think outwardly ... you have altogether a more positive outward focus ... and as *you focus on all the positive aspects of life* it turns out that life ... does it not ... has many exciting surprises?

And soon it will be time to reorient completely to the room/office here with me on [today's date] ... sitting in the chair ... feeling the surface beneath your feet ... fully integrated into the present moment ... with

Ensure that they return to the present moment feeling grounded rather than 'floating around' in a dissociated way

all insights, useful learning, positive thoughts and feelings, every change effected at the unconscious level stored in your reservoir of internal resources so that they will be incorporated naturally and effectively and appropriately into your natural way of thinking, feeling and behaving. Probably you are already becoming more aware of the fabric of the chair ... the feelings in your fingers ... the feeling of the ground/footstool/surface beneath your feet ... confident, positive feelings completely appropriate to the present moment ... you're beginning to see even now in your mind's eye the furniture in the room ... I wonder if you remember exactly what was situated where.

As they have been imagining sexual experience in possibly quite a vivid way, give them plenty of time to adjust to the return to their surroundings in the room/office with you. Bring in allusions to several mundane aspects of their environment before reorienting them completely

Go to a suitable trance reorientation, taking care to remove suggestions of lightness or rigidity of hands that may have been suggested purely for the duration of the trance. However, also take care not to 'suggest back' all normal sensations to the body if 'normal sensations' were perceived as part of the problem. Adding in *Distraction suggestions* may also be useful

Variations, Adaptations and Recommendations to Hypnotic Dreams

A different choice of metaphor can allow the script to be adapted to different personalities and problems. Metaphors more suited to erectile dysfunction and ejaculatory inhibition are included after this script.

Hypnotic dreams

A metaphorical way to encourage women to experience arousal and physical openness.

Dreams are interesting aren't they? ... So many people have had theories about dreams over the years ... wish fulfilment ... a means of sorting out the jigsaw of the day ... a kind of trial run for reality ... a pleasurable fantasy ... metaphorical representations ... sometimes one dream will 'morph' into another one and surprise us ... sometimes our dreams allow us to *do what we really want* when, for whatever reason, our conscious minds had been a bit reluctant ... dreams can let us *find the answer in a metaphor* ... some say that trance is like a waking dream ... others say that trance is what you want it to be at the time ... it's whatever you need it to be to *stimulate your creativity.*

> Pretty much a truism; everybody dreams and many people find them at least vaguely interesting

> Seeds ideas about finding answers in dream metaphors

So whether *you are in a trance* or *you're in a waking dream* at this moment is perhaps just a question of semantics/a choice of words but either way ... it seems to *be an opportunity for something a little different* ... *more openness* to possibilities ... *more* desire to experiment perhaps with this or that idea ... *a flow* of ideas that seem to *come more easily* now.

> Both a trance and a dream are types of altered state

Dreams can be all manner of things to different people ... they can be silky and soft ... they can *be intimate and intriguing* ... they can *be urgent/arousing and powerful* ... they can *be some of these* ... or all of these ... or none of these but *be very seductive* in their own way ... they can be sensational on the surface and deep and meaningful on the inside ... they can be what you want them to be and *their effects can stay with you* long after you have consciously forgotten the dream itself ... but *there's something inside that remembers ... and stirs.*

> Use your voice to emphasize appropriate embedded commands

I wonder what the theorists make of the flower dream … I love those secretive yet wonderfully responsive flowers that … when the sun comes out … *open up and seem to reach out* for the warmth and light of the sun … other people *like the sun-flower that stands tall and proud* with vibrant colour and passion … yet others *love the white snow flow-ers that are usually the first to push through* the win-ter ground and *delight us when we see them* … and then there's the rose with its perfume … sometimes delicate and sometimes sultry … the rose with its tight bud that can *show such a different side* when we see it in full bloom.

Metaphors for opening or pushing through

Talking of dreams … did you know that you can program your dreams? When you go to bed … you can begin to daydream the dream you want to have … *let it be colourful … and full of pleasurable experi-ences that appeal to all your senses* … and *your unconscious* … that *knows how to do this* … can bring that dream back to you in the night or in the early morning … can *let your whole self feel the sen-sation* … a waking dream can turn into a sleeping dream at night … and a warm … moist … intensely pleasurable sensation that makes itself felt in a spe-cial way can … in turn … evoke a waking dream again … and *(a)rouse you and allow the fantasy to continue in the most exquisite way* … maybe an unexpected wakeful way … maybe waking and sur-prising that person beside you … which of you is the more surprised, I wonder … and delighted … could this be what people mean by 'living the dream'?

You really can program your dreams

The dream may allow you to experience the sensation. Your unconscious knows how to do it

Additional metaphors

I wonder what the theorists make of the 'brain-body scan' dream ... you know how these days it's possible to scan the brain using special imaging techniques to see which areas of the brain are active ... they light up in different colours according to the type of thought ... and in this dream you can actually watch as a thought appears in the brain ... in colours ... and shapes ... moving in ever changing patterns ... and then you search around the body to see where the thought in the brain *stirs the response in the body* ... and *one response triggers another and then another* ... as different parts light up ... and people find that ... *as soon as they enter* the scanner that *they can increase the intensity of the activity* ... the colours can *become more vital and vibrant* ... the shapes and patterns change and pulsate ... some people *become very inventive* as they *deliberately intensify the fantasy or see an image or feel a touch* and see the brain activity change *instantly* and direct their amazing hormonal messengers with the speed of lighting to *light up the body.*

Metaphors for thoughts and images to light up parts of the body and stir a response. Could be useful for increasing desire in either men or women

* * *

I wonder what the theorists would make of a fountain dream I heard of ... there are all kinds of fountain dreams ... but this interesting dream was inspired by a trip to Hellbrunn Castle in Austria ... there are many castles in Austria ... each *with a different feeling* about it ... but this castle has trick fountains in the gardens ... with *jets of water* that *can be turned on at will* ... all done by internal water pressure and plumbing ... visitors walk around the gardens *admiring the view* when suddenly *they are surprised/soaked* by a jet of water ... and in his dream this man became the fountain operator and *took intense pleasure in spraying/squirting jets of water at what he thought was just the right moment.*

This metaphor is primarily for ejaculatory inhibition but the emphasis could also be placed on the strength and force of the fountain and so make it more of an analogy for an erection

'turned on at will' **suggests control**

Letting go of inhibition

This script would be suitable for a woman who feels inhibited about experiencing sexual desire or pleasure. It would not be appropriate for somebody who had suffered abuse or a traumatic sexual experience so take a full case history to establish that this is not the cause of the problem. Even in such a case, however, extracts of the script could usefully be very carefully adapted and made use of at a later stage in treatment.

Have you ever noticed that people can spend an enormous amount of time and energy searching for answers to problems … they tie themselves up in knots … going round and round and over and over … making things more and more complex … sometimes they get stuck in blaming themselves … or blaming other people … and still don't come up with an answer … and somehow it doesn't occur to them to look for something simple … and yet very often that is indeed the best answer of all.

Sometimes I think this is the way it is with sexual issues … just think for a moment about how so many people pick up/develop attitudes and feelings about sex when they were quite young … maybe at a time when … although their bodies were mature, their minds hadn't quite caught up … they hadn't given themselves time to fully develop their own thoughts and attitudes … so they accepted other people's attitudes at the unconscious level … even without knowing that this was what they were doing.

Consider the young girl for example who experiments with sex … under pressure to please someone … under pressure from her peers … or under pressure from her own physical/urge/strength of feeling … so she goes along with what is wanted or expected but at the same time she has the feeling that it's wrong or that it's dirty … or that it's against her personal standards and this thought sticks so that later on … long after she is old enough to make her own decisions … and form her own opinions

It could be that she has internalised parental or religious values that are not appropriate in her current situation or stage in life

91

... she has taken on/internalised the thought that she shouldn't really enjoy this because it's dirty/it's shameful/it's not allowed ... and so denies herself a pleasure that should be hers.

And there could be a very simple answer ... take a moment to understand ... that now you are a grown woman ... you can make your own decisions that can be wise and generous ... you can give yourself permission to *be yourself and enjoy yourself* ... *enjoy your emotions ... your thoughts and your body* ... have a look inside yourself for the part inside you that has been withholding permission for you to enjoy sensual pleasure ... check it out ... where did that come from? ... Was it from a time when different standards applied? ... Was it from a parent? ... Was it from a belief that was right then but not now? ...Was it from a standard that was appropriate for a child but not for an adult? ... Take all the time you need to go through that in your mind and when you have decided that the choice lies with you and nobody else, you can realise that however complex the origins of that decision ... that the answer can be very simple ... you can *give yourself permission to take a pleasure in the sexual act now that it is the right stage in your life*/you are with the right person for you ... it is *your* body and it is *your* decision and it is *your* permission to give yourself whenever you're ready ... take all the time you want and let me know once you've done whatever you need to do today ... knowing that you are capable of very wise instinctive responses that can impact on you in a very positive way. [Pause] And in a few moments you will begin that process of reorientation and at some inner level your mind and your body will become aware of this positive impact and look forward to the awareness of your outer self that will inevitably follow in forthcoming days and weeks.

Recommended reorientation: *Unconscious continuation*

Simple can sound appealing

Add in anything that you think will resonate with your client

Essential Tremor

Considerations

Only treat patients after a medical diagnosis of Essential Tremor, also known as Benign Tremor, and with the agreement of a medical practitioner. It shares some symptoms with other serious neurological disorders such as Parkinson's disease and it is diagnosed only after any other possible cause has been ruled out. It is therefore of crucial importance to have the tremor medically investigated, diagnosed and appropriately treated.

To date (2010), and to the best of my knowledge, no scientific studies have demonstrated the effectiveness of hypnosis in treating Essential Tremor but, anecdotally, patients have reported an improvement in their observations and feelings of calm and control over the tremor.

Essential Tremor is a neurological disorder which can affect almost any part of the body, and also the voice, but it commonly occurs in the hands, arms or head. It is characterised by a trembling which is most evident during simple motor tasks such as eating and drinking, writing, applying make-up or shaving. It becomes more prevalent with age although it can also occur in younger patients.

Many patients will report that it worsens with anxiety and stress so individually relevant suggestions for dealing with these factors should always be included in treatment and a progressive relaxation would be a good choice of induction. In addition to general stress and anxiety it should be remembered that the condition itself can cause sufferers a considerable amount of embarrassment, irritation and annoyance, sometimes grief over loss of former good health and worries about what the future may hold.

The use of a hand levitation (or a cataleptic hand induction) in *Reinforce and intensify changes achieved* is particularly apt because it demonstrates the power of the unconscious mind over a limb. However, since the levitation normally produces shaky movements, do NOT choose the affected hand or arm for this process. In this instance it has been selected for use in a later or final treatment session as a means of ratifying progress and giving reassurance that progress will be continued and sustained. A good argument could equally be made for using such a powerful and convincing induction in a first treatment session.

Variations, Adaptations and Recommendations

The following scripts have been designed as a set of three consecutive treatment sessions, each building on the last. They can, however, be used independently with only minor adaptation, or omission of certain phrases. Use an *induction/deepener* to achieve deep relaxation with the first script. The second script revivifies previous trance experience. The third script includes a hand levitation induction *for use with the unaffected hand*.

In addition to the scripts in this section, you can select and adapt scripts in the *Vocal and motor tics* section. This could be useful if the patient does not perceive any immediate benefit from *Calm and steady the hand and arm*. The script *Regain ease of movement and control* is intended for use after there has been noticeable improvement in calming the tremor itself. The *Surgery and recovery of health* section also contains scripts for healing that can be adapted for use. The *Anxiety, Panic and Phobias* section contains scripts or script extracts that you may find useful for dealing with any accompanying stress.

Calm and steady the hand and arm

Here in this calm and relaxed hypnotic state I invite you to make full use of both parts of your mind ... your conscious and *your unconscious*. You probably already know that your unconscious mind is the part of you that controls your autonomic bodily functions ... controls your breathing and your blood flow and also controls the unconscious movements in your body ... and here ... it's good to know that this relaxed state of mind will greatly enhance channels of communication between the two parts of the mind and also ensure a positive outcome.

So just take a moment or two to use your conscious mind to ask *your unconscious* for its help to *take more and more control of the fingers ... take more and more control of the hand and take more and more control of the arm* ... in a way that it can *become steadier and still* whenever you want it to ... wherever you want it to *relax and calm right down* and *feel more comfortable in every way* ... just ask it mentally and silently to help now in the process today and nod your head when you've done it. [*Pause*] Excellent. Thank you.

Now normally of course ... you may never have noticed exactly how or where you naturally *take control of all movement ... even microscopic movement in your body ... but* each of us has a way to do this through unconscious communication between brain and body ... and with the help that your unconscious mind has agreed to give you today ... you can go inside and *look for the control centre inside you.* ... Some people will find switches that can be flicked on or off to *take control* ... and others will *find a control* that you *can reach out and turn down* ... a bit like an old volume control where you turn it round to *turn it down or turn it off* ... and some people will find a key pad ... just like the ones on a remote control ... that you press to lessen the volume or

Hypnosis is a state that involves both a conscious and unconscious process

'Your unconscious' is emphasised with the voice to exploit ambiguity (You're unconscious). This also has the effect of encouraging dissociation

Embedded commands for control

This section gives suggestions for imagery, but also gives the client permission to use the particular imagery appropriate to them. It also includes embedded commands for control

change the TV channel ... whatever you find will be perfect for you.

So now in your mind's eye ... I'd like you to see that hand and that arm and notice how you can *adjust your inner control right now ... and calm down that shaking/trembling/jerky movement* ... turn it right down so it becomes steadier and steadier ... steadier and steadier ... steadier and steadier still ... and let me know when you see it becoming completely still. [Pause] That's it.

Use the words the patient has used to describe the tremor

Good. Now have another look at that mental image of the hand and arm ... this time just beginning to shake slightly ... and I'd like you to look at it and tell it to 'Calm down/Settle down right now/Stop' ... or use whichever words seem the right ones for you ... and as you *give it that instruction very firmly*, watch the hand and feel the hand quietening down ... calming down ... becoming steady ... becoming perfectly still ... and let me know when you've done it. [Pause]

Bring in all the senses, visual, auditory and kinaesthetic (VAK) to make it a richer experience

The more often you do this mental exercise, the more *easily* this calming, steadying process will happen ... the more often you do this, the more *naturally* it will happen ... the more often you do this, the more *automatically* it will happen. So just before we finish the session today ... I invite you to *go over this exercise in your mind in every tiny little detail* in the situations where the tremor *used to happen* in your daily life ... *seeing the calming process* happening as soon as you *give yourself the instruction* ... *hearing your own words inside* ... *feeling* the calming and steadying occurring ... until you *become so comfortable* with this response, *it has become automatic* ... so you will find in your daily life that any time you get a sense of unsteadiness beginning ... all you have to do is to look at the hand ... mentally give it your instruction and then enjoy watching as you feel it becoming more and more steady ... more and more calm ... becoming more and more still. And

Linked direct commands

Repetition of imagery of taking control in their everyday situations will strengthen the desired response

Note the change of tense *'it has become automatic'*

isn't it fascinating to *notice how your mind is now taking control* at both the conscious and unconscious level and how *this will continue long after this session is over.*

And in a few moments time you will feel an urge to reorient to the room ... increase your sense of wakeful alertness and awareness of calm control of every part of your body ... each day this sense of hopeful positivity in you will be refreshed as you practise this mental exercise and notice the physical effects more and more each day. And I'm wondering ... which aspects of all this new-found control will be the most encouraging ... the most satisfying ... the most surprising over the *days and weeks ahead ... as perhaps you are wondering too?* And by the way ... I'd like to congratulate you on your ability here today to find the depth of relaxation and ease of communication between conscious and unconscious minds and body ... and let you know that this experience today allows you to achieve that state even more swiftly ... even more deeply whenever you want to achieve it again.

People like to be reassured they have done well

Post-hypnotic suggestion for subsequent swift achievement of the state

Go to a suitable trance reorientation. NB It is very important NOT to suggest back symptoms in the reorientation stage so take care to omit common phrases such as 'all normal sensations will return to the body'

Regain ease of movement and control

This script is suitable for use on a second visit *after there has already been some success with steadying the trembling in the limb*. The script addresses the restricted movement and partial loss of control and strength which frequently accompanies Essential Tremor. It can be useful to demonstrate the power of suggestion and visualisation by asking the patient to carry out a desired action, such as retrieving something from a back pocket or using a knife and fork, before the trance state and then again afterwards to notice the improvement.

And as you allow your eyes to close ... settling yourself down and finding the most comfortable position for you ... letting the muscles in your body relax ... mentally scanning your body to discover where and how your body likes to relax first ... feeling the comfort and ease and noticing the support beneath your head ... your neck ... your shoulders ... your back ... your arms ... down into your hands and your fingers ... you may be finding that just *the sound of the voice is already bringing back familiar feelings of calm and ease and relaxation* from the last time you relaxed so comfortably here ... even already being reminded of the enhanced communication of the conscious and unconscious parts of your mind ... and how delightful is it to realise ... now you know just how good it feels to *relax so deeply* ... that you have the ability to *relax even more swiftly* than before ... *relax even more completely* than before ... *relax even more profoundly* than before ... all through the body ... the chest ... the trunk of your body ... down into your legs and all the way down to your feet ... wonderful.

Revivifies thoughts and feelings from previous trance state

Evokes the post-hypnotic suggestion from the previous script *Calm and steady the hand and arm* if it was used

And as you relax so pleasantly ... I'd like to congratulate you on the differences you have experienced since I saw you last ... how interesting it was for you to notice how that hand/arm was able to *achieve a sense of steadiness and calm* ... seemingly all on its own but really with the help of *your unconscious* mind ... a powerful partnership between your conscious and your unconscious mind ... as you consciously

Comment on any specific positive changes reported in your pre-trance discussion thus ratifying and reinforcing responses. This also gives more opportunity for embedded commands

Encourages control at both the conscious and unconscious level

*remembere*d to look at the arm/hand and give it the simple, firm instruction to *'Calm down/Settle down right now/Stop'* and *your unconscious* mind had the power to *make it happen/carry it out.*

Today we are going to *strengthen that response* and add a few new ones as well … so in a moment … I'm going to ask you to … mentally and silently … send some messages to the part of *your uncon-scious* mind that controls your movements … some people will *see a clear picture of themselves carry-ing out this action* … some people will *get a fleeting sense/impression of its happening* … some people will *sense their muscles moving* as they mentally *talk themselves through the actions* … some people *have a very rich experience of seeing … and hear-ing … and feeling everything happening just as it should … whichever way you experience this will be perfect for you … Now you might like to con-sider these messages …* 'I want to *move* my *arm decisively behind* me and firmly *reach into* my *back pocket with* my *hand.'* [Pause] *'I will grasp the wallet with my fingers and grip it strongly.'* [Pause] *'I will pull it out firmly and easily.'* [Pause] And notice how your unconscious mind will let you *fully experience a sense of this happening right now … and you may have some other messages that you would like to send before we move on … take all the time you need.* [Pause]

Bringing in all the senses enriches the experience and, phrased in this way, it also removes pressure from those people who claim not to be able to visualise well

Use actions selected beforehand by your patient. Leave pauses after each instruction for the patient to relay the message to their unconscious mind

You may already know … or you may be hearing it now as completely new information … that experi-ments have been performed that show that people who *practise doing something in perfect detail in their minds,* dramatically increase their ability to carry it out in their daily lives … and the more often you do this in your imagination, *the better you will perform these actions each and every day …* so let's go through it again right now … pay attention to every little detail and be sure you make everything happen exactly as you want it to do right now … after all … this is *your* mind and *your* imagination so you can

Gives the rationale for repetition of the visualisation

make/have it happen perfectly … so, see it in your mind's eye or just get that sense of it happening and … be there now, feeling every movement so decisive and steady and firm and notice how you can … so easily … extend your arm further than you could before … hearing yourself on the inside giving yourself any necessary instructions which ensure you carry it out with ease … nod your head once you've done this to your satisfaction. [Pause] Well done.

VAK

Now just before we move on/bring the session to a close, I invite you to consider if there is still any possible improvement you can make … to *make that performance as perfect as you want it to be* … perhaps you can *do it a little quicker … or do it with a little more ease and dexterity … or do it with a little more precision … if so,* just add that in now and *feel it in your arm … feel it in your hand and feel it in your fingers as you experience it just as you want it to be … do it now* and you will hear my voice reassuring and reinforcing as you *do it right now.*

Pre-warns that the end of the activity or the session is in sight which has the effect of concentrating the mind and possibly increasing receptivity to suggestion

While they carry out this visualisation, you can very softly encourage as appropriate; Good, Good job, That's right, Yes, You can do this so well etc.

The more often you do this visualisation in your mind at home, the more easily it will happen in your body … the more often you do this, the more *naturally* this will happen … the more often you do this, the more *automatically* this will happen. So have a think now about the best *times and places where you can … stop … and take a couple of minutes to run through this simple activity in your mind in every tiny little detail* … perhaps in the morning before you get up … at night before you go to sleep is a very good time … mid-morning and after lunch … until you *become so comfortable and familiar with this ease of movement that it has become second nature to you.*

Suggests the value of regular practice and gives the opportunity to reflect on suitable times for them

And as the days and the weeks and the months go by, you will *steadily* find that you *internalise this response/these responses so powerfully and effectively,* it/they will be occurring just as a natural part of your life … as natural as breathing … as natural as sleeping … as natural as speaking … just a natural part of you.

Choose a different suggestion if breathing, sleeping or speaking are associated with problems

And in a few moments time I am going to suggest that you begin that process of reorienting to the room when you will increase your sense of wakeful alertness and you will experience a wonderful feeling of renewal of hope … a sense of enthusiasm and eagerness to build on your success … and of course you know that this positive, hopeful outlook will be refreshed as you practise this mental exercise and notice the physical effects more and more each day. And I'm wondering … which aspects of all this new-found control will be the most pleasing … the most satisfying … the most surprising over the *days and weeks ahead … as perhaps you are wondering too?*

Go to a suitable trance reorientation. NB It is very important NOT to suggest back symptoms in the reorientation stage so take care to omit common phrases such as 'all normal sensations will return to the body'

Reinforce and intensify changes achieved

The hand levitation induction included here is for use with the hand and arm that is strong and completely unaffected by tremor. It is unsuitable where both hands are affected by a tremor.

Demonstrate the appropriate positioning of hands. Have the palm of the unaffected hand facing downwards, the fingers barely touching the knees, the palm slightly raised and without the arm or elbow being supported in any way, thus easing the process of levitation. The other hand should rest comfortably and heavily on the lap.

It is essential to have the patient focus on the hand unaffected by tremor.

I'd like you to rest your fingertips very, very lightly on your knees ... that's right ... just like this ... your fingertips barely touching and focus your attention on that hand ... focus all your attention on the hand ... that's right and just listening to the sound of my voice that you already know relaxes you and enables you to *achieve that wonderful trance state* ... I'd like you to *become very aware of the changes you observe in the hand* ... can you notice how ... as you look at the hand ... you may *find changes beginning to happen?* ... It may seem to you that *the hand is becoming fuzzy and blurred* ... yes, fuzzy and blurred ... or it may be that the opposite happens ... *you may notice a very defined outline around the hand* ... becoming more and more defined ... interesting ... yes, very interesting to *notice these things* and allow yourself to *experience them fully* ... in whatever way they occur ... for it may be that you *first experience the visual changes* ... or it may be that first of all ... as you turn your attention now to the weight of the hand ... (*or is it lightness?*) ... there is an experience of that *hand feeling lighter and lighter* ... the more you *focus your attention on the sensations in the hand, the more apparent those changes seem to be* ... in fact ... can you *notice the slight tingling in the fingertips?* ... Notice any little movement ... any little lifting urge ... becoming aware of that *lifting*

Direct the patient's focus on to the NON-tremor hand

Use a light, interested, questioning tone of voice and leave plenty of pauses for changes to be observed

'*The* or *that* hand' encourages dissociation

You can allow your own hand to lift very slightly so that the patient will notice this *only in their peripheral vision*. This reinforces the suggestions of lightness and lifting at the unconscious level

urge in perhaps one finger ... or is it in more than one finger? ... Or is it *the thumb first* that is wanting to lift higher and higher? ... Or is it *all the fingers* ... as the lightness spreads back into the knuckles? ... And is the whole hand now feeling lighter ... with the urge to *lift higher and higher becoming irresistible* ... as if the hand has a mind of its own? ... as if it can decide all by itself that it *will* lift higher *and higher* as if it's floating ... as indeed it *can* float ... *all on its own* ... *higher and higher* ... *all on its own at the unconscious level.*

The suggestions allow a variety of response

Reinforce any quiver/slight movement with a comment such as 'Yes, That's right, Interesting'

'float ... *all on its own*' *encourages* dissociation

And as you continue to observe the hand floating and lifting all on its own ... you may also become aware of the feeling of heaviness in your other hand as it rests so calmly there ... how, as the one hand gets lighter and lighter ... the other becomes heavier and yet more still and yet more calm ... just as you can notice that heaviness is developing in your eyelids ... heavier and heavier in your eyelids ... as the urge for them to close becomes more insistent now ... that's right ... allowing that wonderful sense of relief to spread over you as the eyelids close and you develop that deeper sense of hypnotic relaxation.

Shifts attention to the steadiness and heaviness of the other hand

Suggestions for heavy eyelids are more effective if synchronised with the patient's blinking response

And as you allow this deepening to occur I invite you to consider the power of your unconscious mind in taking control of the movement of the hand and the arm ... how amazing it is ... [Pause] and I'm going to suggest that your unconscious continues its excellent work on your behalf over the forthcoming days and weeks ... days and weeks turning into months and years of steady and sustained progress. Take the time once again with your conscious mind to reassure your unconscious mind that you are completely happy for it to find the right way for you to *calm and steady your arm and hand more and more each day ... this is what you want for you ...* that's right.

This phrase ostensibly refers to the control of the *floating hand* but can also refer to the control of the *previously trembling hand*

Not only progress but *sustained* progress

So in a few moments time you will find that ... as soon as your unconscious is ready to *accept responsibility for continuing calm and control of the left/right hand* ... the floating hand will begin to float downwards and back to your lap ... all the while regaining its normal weight as it drifts downward ... that's it ... interesting ... your unconscious seems delighted to accept responsibility ... for increasing *calm and steadiness* ... good ... increasing flexibility ... extending range of movement ... letting go of any possible vestige of tension ... feeling now this sense of calm and tranquillity spreading all the way down from your neck and into your shoulders ... noticing perhaps a sense of ease spreading all the way down from your shoulders into your arms ... and then ... deeper and deeper relaxed ... and now all the way down into your wrists and into your hands ... steady and still ... still and steady ... yes, all the way down ... that's right.

Select *left or right hand* **as appropriate. Avoid mentioning the tremor so as not to suggest it back again**

The acknowledgement of downward movements of the hand attribute responsibility to the unconscious mind

And ... here in this heightened state of communication ... your conscious mind, your unconscious mind and your body ... are working together in harmony once again to *carry out all the calm and control you need for positive functioning...* so that from now on you will be able to *keep steady control of your hand and arm* ... you will be able to *move your arm with increasing ease* ... you will find that as you use it more, *your grip becomes firmer and firmer ... and what is more ... you will be noticing a sense of calm that is not only in your arm and hand ... you* are handling everything in your daily life more easily and calmly than before ... sometimes even finding it a little curious to think ... if you bother to think about it at all ... that once you *used to* perceive certain things as a bit stressful ... for now you take those things in your stride as of no consequence at all ... just as normal everyday aspects of life ... and it seems that now you have a zest for life which is stronger than ever before.

Post-hypnotic suggestions

So now in your mind's eye ... I'd like you to see yourself in a mental film over the next few days and weeks carrying out your normal everyday activities

… noticing every detail … making more and more progress … noticing how … should you ever need to … you can look at your arm/hand and give it your command 'Settle down right now' … *hearing your own words inside* as you feel yourself *adjusting that inner control … directing a little more calm to wherever you want it … a little more control whenever you want it* so it becomes steadier and steadier … steadier and steadier … steadier and steadier still … that's it … perfectly still. But also when you need to use it … look at how your hand is grasping and gripping more firmly than you've done in a long time and … as you practise … that grip is getting firmer and firmer … *feeling* it happen until you *become so comfortable* with this response that it will *continue automatically … becoming steadier and stronger with each passing day.*

Bringing in all the senses increases the intensity of the experience

And in a few moments … you will begin to notice a sense of eagerness to return to more wakeful alertness and a feeling of being refreshed … with renewed energy and vitality … each day this sense of vitality will be refreshed as you continue to practise this mental visualisation and notice the positive effect on you. And I'm wondering … who else will be noticing something different in you … which aspects will they see … will it be the physical changes or will it be some indefinable lifting of spirits over the *days and weeks ahead?*

Directs focus outwards

Go to a suitable trance reorientation with suggestions for removal of *inappropriate* lightness or heaviness, particularly mentioning the limbs and eyelids referred to in the induction. NB It is very important NOT to suggest back symptoms in the reorientation stage so take care to omit common phrases such as 'all normal sensations will return to the body'

Vocal and Motor Tics

Considerations and aims

- Tics are classified as a neurological disorder under the heading of dyskinesia, which means abnormal involuntary movements. There is often no known cause. Research on biological, chemical and environmental factors continues.
- Tics usually begin in childhood, although there is evidence of rare cases of new onset in adults. More detailed questioning often reveals that tics had been present transiently in childhood but had reduced or disappeared for several, if not many, years.
- There is some evidence to suggest that these rare cases of sudden onset tics in adults may be triggered by encephalitis, recreational drug use, certain prescription medication, head trauma or streptococcal infection.
- Tics diagnosed as transient will usually have disappeared by adulthood and those diagnosed as chronic are the ones which may continue into adulthood.
- They may appear singly or in clusters and may worsen with stress, excitement, fatigue or illness although they are not caused by anxiety. They may be simple, single sounds or movements involving a single set of muscle groups or they may be complex, sequences of movements involving different muscle groups or sounds. The complexity may even result in little steps or routines more like dance movements.
- The tics are sometimes mild and sometimes frighteningly forceful.
- Although tics are involuntary, they sometimes can be controlled or suppressed with a great deal of effort and associated tension.
- They are often found to coexist in ADHD or OCD sufferers.
- Children and adults suffering with tic disorder are thought to be more at risk of depression, probably as a result of coping with the problem and social withdrawal.
- Tics are thought to be on a spectrum with the mildest of transient tics on the one side and the most severe Tourette's syndrome on the other.
- Medication is the most common form of treatment, but there is as yet no cure.
- Behavioural programmes have been found helpful in reduction of tics and in coping more easily emotionally.

General aims for hypnotherapy

- Increase calm and relaxation in general.
- Take control over the tic in specific places/specific occasions/ for longer periods without increasing associated tension. (Agree times and places to release tension through free expression of their tics.)
- Become aware of signs that the tic is about to occur and install triggers for control of the tic at this stage.
- Change perception of the tic from overwhelming to manageable.
- Build confidence and self-esteem.
- Cope with embarrassment and other people's responses.
- Encourage them to feel able to explain the problem to others without embarrassment or shame.
- Deal with possible related problems such as OCD or ADHD.

Useful approaches and techniques

- Focus, distraction or relaxation inductions.
- Direct suggestions for calm and control.
- Metaphor that allows a sense of control and manipulation of the symptom.
- Guided visualisation of successful management of the tic.

Another approach, which at first sight flies in the face of medical opinion, is to assume that the tic was triggered by an emotional response and to regress the patient to that time and allow cathartic release of a suppressed emotion and so have no emotional need for the tic response. Parts work could also be used to release the need for the response. On reflection this may not be as out of line with medical thinking as it at first sounds. If we assume that the individual may have a genetic propensity for tics and we recognize that stress plays a part in worsening the condition, and we further know that relaxation and a calm emotional state can improve the condition, is it beyond the bounds of possibility that extreme emotional trauma can trigger the onset of a tic in someone with a propensity for such behaviour? I can only cite my own experience in working with certain clients where almost all symptoms seemed to disappear after such treatment. Using a computer metaphor or a master control room where the symptoms can be manipulated has also proved effective.

Your body knows how to let the tic rest and sleep

Some tics subside during periods of rest and sleep. Before assuming that this is the case you need to check it out with any individual client. 'Talking to the part that knows how to do this' allows this ability to be mapped across to waking situations.

And in this comfortable hypnotic relaxation ... it's the ideal time to *make contact with the innermost parts of you* that are particularly attentive and open to communication in this state ... now you know that there is a part of you that lets the tic rest (completely) when you relax and sleep ... and during that time, *the tic is completely calm and comfortable as it sleeps* while you yourself sleep ... so I suggest that you have a conversation right now with that part and ask it to *allow that tic to spend more and more time resting and sleeping* even while you yourself are wide awake and getting on with your life ... explain all the benefits that this will give you in your life. [Pause] Now you may even find that you *receive a signal somewhere in your body ... a sensation ... or hear a 'yes' in your mind* ... some people *do* ... *get that internal signal* that lets you *know that you have reached agreement at the innermost level to let that tic spend more and more time enjoying resting and sleeping* even though you yourself are wide awake and getting on with your everyday activities ... or indeed all of this agreement may be entirely at the unconscious level ... whichever way, I invite you to spend some time now going over in great detail in your mind ... just like having a deliberate daydream ... exactly how *things are going to be more comfortable for you* now that the tic has decided to spend so much more time ... or perhaps all of its time ... asleep and comfortable ... allowing you to get on with enjoying your everyday life. ... Use all of your senses ... use your eyes to *see how you look so much more at ease* and are calmly getting on with your life with fewer interruptions ... hardly aware of those movements/sounds at all ... use your feelings to *feel that degree of calm and control* you are

Reframes the truism that there are times when the tic is less apparent during sleep

A way of reclaiming some control over an unconscious response

Offers many possibilities of response which are all acceptable

Reassures them that even without a conscious signal this is fine, because it may happen entirely at the unconscious level

Presupposition that things will be more comfortable, the question is how it will manifest itself

Use all the senses VAK

experiencing now … use your ears to *hear how life is more peaceful and calm* … use every part of you to *intensify this experience of peace and calm and control at both inner and outer levels and when you have finished this … and please do take all the time you want … you can let me know.*

Include other therapeutic suggestions, give ego strengthening or go to a suitable trance reorientation

Variations, Adaptations and Recommendations

Where tics do not subside during relaxation or sleep, they may in fact do so during periods of intense activity or concentration such as sport or working on the computer. In this case, adapt the script by talking to the part that knows how to let the tic rest and sleep in those situations and negotiate as above.

Explain away embarrassment

The script aims to help deal with associated embarrassment of tics. You can 'borrow' this true story about blushing or change it to 'someone I know used to be a champion blusher'. There are several advantages to using a story or metaphor such as this: it gives an example of a fellow sufferer's success which can gain rapport and can also be inspiring; it also gives an opportunity to deliver embedded commands to the client in quotes, which are ostensibly directed towards somebody else. This may have the effect of by-passing conscious resistance from the client.

Many years ago I used to be a champion blusher ... I was exceptionally good at it ... I could blush for seemingly no reason at all ... I could blush redder and brighter than anyone I ever knew ... I could even be by myself and think about the possibility of blushing, and I would blush then and there all on my own ... sometimes quite spectacularly. ... the worst thing about it for me was worrying that people would notice ... and then one day somebody gave me a tip and *that simple tip just took all the worry away* ... funny, ... isn't it? ... how complex problems don't always need complex solutions ... simple ones will do very well ... this man told me that he *used* to have a tic and *used* to feel embarrassed ... hoping that people wouldn't notice and one day he just decided to be the first to remark on it ... he would say, 'Oh, by the way, I have a bit of a tic where I might clear my throat/jerk my arm/blink my eyes/ twitch my nose' so that from thereon in he could just *stop worrying about it* ... he could just *stop feeling awkward* about it ... he told me the best thing to do was to *ignore it* ... 'that's what I do' he said ... 'and then *you can forget about it* ... and *pretty soon you'll be hardly aware of it at all* as it just *disappears calmly and quietly all on its own.*' ... And you know, I took his advice ... I explained to people that sometimes I blushed for seemingly no reason at all and the best thing for them to do was the same thing that I did ... *just ignore it* ... and you know what ... I really did

The first part of the metaphor carries a similarity to the problem of a tic but is not the identical problem

Worry about others' reactions can sometimes exacerbate the tic

Use your voice to emphasise the words 'used to'

Success story of fellow sufferer can be motivating

Embedded commands throughout this next section

explain away the problem so I was able to *forget about it* and gradually, over a period of time … it forgot about itself most of the time … so that now … if it were to happen at all … *it's a matter of complete indifference … has absolutely no significance at all.*

Although the script is designed to cope with embarrassment, the final suggestion is aimed at the tic itself. The phrase 'if it were to happen at all' **lends doubt to the recurrence**

Variations, Adaptations and Recommendations

Naturally, you could also use this script for blushing itself adding in other suggestions for dealing with particular triggering situations.

Tic script extracts – calm a premonitory urge

Various suggestions which could be included in scripts as appropriate to symptom and the individual.

Some sufferers are aware of a 'premonitory urge' immediately prior to the onset of a tic. These localised sensations are variously described by sufferers: a build up of tension similar to the need to sneeze or scratch an itch, a sense of discomfort with a strong urge to blink, to clear the throat, to shrug the shoulders. A couple of examples have been given and can be adapted to suit the specific tic to be eliminated or reduced.

The urge to blink

As soon as you notice the build-up of sensation/feeling/discomfort in your eye you will find yourself saying the word *'calm'* to yourself and a wonderful feeling of calm will spread all over your face and all over your body and *that old urge to blink will fade right away … right now … that's right …* At first, you will actually say the word *'calm'* and … *as you say the word 'calm' the feelings will subside/calm down/fade away/disappear and you will feel completely relaxed. …* I wonder how soon it will be before you will only need to *say the word 'calm' silently in your head and the feelings will fade right away …* right there and then … and *there will be absolutely no urge to blink …* and as the days and the weeks and the months go by … you will find more and more that … just *as soon as you begin to notice that build-up of sensation … the urge will disappear automatically …* the sensation itself has become a trigger for the urge to *disappear completely … the urge will disappear completely.*

Post-hypnotic suggestion

Presupposition that this will occur. The emphasis has changed to *how soon* it will happen. Also serves to build positive expectation for the future

Post-hypnotic suggestion and reframe of the premonitory urge itself as a signal for the tic to disappear

The urge to clear the throat

As soon as you notice the sensation/feeling/dis-comfort in your throat you will find yourself thinking the word '*calm*' and a wonderful feeling of calm and comfort will spread all over your face, your neck and all through your throat … all the muscles in your mouth and throat will relax and *that old urge to clear the throat will relax away … right away* … right now … that's right … at first, you will deliberately think the word '*calm*' and as you *hear the word 'calm' in your head … the feelings will relax right away* … and *you will feel completely relaxed* … and *there will be a wonderful feeling of calm in your throat* … com-pletely at ease … completely calm … I wonder how soon it will be before *you notice that you no longer even have to think the word calm … because the merest hint of sensation in your throat has automati-cally become the trigger/signal for the urge to relax away* … right away … right there and then … and as the days and the weeks and the months go by … you will find more and more that … *the urge will disappear* completely … *the urge will have disap-peared completely.*

Post-hypnotic suggestion

The premonitory urge itself becomes a signal for the tic to disappear

Variations, Adaptations and Recommendations

Instead of using the auditory anchor 'calm' you could suggest a physical gesture, a squeeze of the fingers or touch on an incon-spicuous part of the body.

Irritable Bowel Syndrome (IBS)

Considerations

Check that patients suffering from the various symptoms of IBS have a medical diagnosis as some of the symptoms are shared by more serious conditions.

It is usually diagnosed by ruling out all other conditions such as colon cancer, Crohn's disease or ulcerative colitis.

IBS has a collection of symptoms which vary greatly in severity from person to person and not all symptoms are present with every patient. It is more frequently found in women and symptoms are often reported to worsen around menstruation time. Many people find that symptoms are worsened by particular foods whereas in others this seems not to be an issue.

Stress certainly aggravates IBS although it doesn't cause it. Suffering from the condition itself can cause a great deal of stress and anxiety and, in some cases, can negatively affect many areas of life, even occasionally causing people to change their job or leave work altogether.

Patients with IBS have a tendency to be more focused on and sensitive to abdominal sensation than those without it. Symptoms may be relatively mild or so severe that patients find it difficult to leave environments they consider 'safe'. Some suffer from travel toilet phobia and refuse to travel without knowing the exact location of public toilets throughout their entire proposed journey. Merely being in possession of this information is sufficient for some people not to require them whereas others will genuinely need to make use of toilet facilities several times in a relatively short space of time.

Hypnotherapy has a very good track record in dealing with this problem and clinics exist in certain hospitals where hypnotherapy is offered, often as a first line of treatment.

Common symptoms include:

- Abdominal bloating
- Abdominal pain and cramping
- Flatulence (gas)
- Diarrhoea or constipation, or both alternately
- Feelings of incomplete evacuation even after having a bowel movement.

In addition to the scripts given here, some of those in the following sections will be found useful:

- *Coping with pain*
- *Surgery and recovery of health*
- *Anxiety, Panic, Phobias,* notably *Travel toilet phobia.*

The scripts dealing with urinary problems could also be adapted and made use of in some instances.

Relaxation of the digestive tract

Use the *Mental massage* script as an induction.

And can you *notice now* ... *really* notice ... how ... as all of those wonderful feelings of comfort and calm have been spreading through the body ... the amazing feeling of pure relaxation seems to spread all through the muscles and nerves in your entire body ... the *internal* organs have been relaxing too ... on the inside ... all the way through your entire digestive tract the muscles and nerves are relaxing ... feel how your throat is calm and relaxed ... feel all the muscles and nerves in your oesophagus relaxing all the way down that long passage way to the stomach ... feeling so calm and relaxed ... relaxation spreading right through the trunk of your body ... the stomach is calm and relaxed and carrying out all its normal functions with such ease and comfort ... all the muscles and nerves in the small intestine relaxing ... that's right ... that's it ... a chain reaction of amazing calm and comfort ... now spreading into the colon ... calm and comfort ... easily and effortlessly ... spreading all through the twists and turns of the intestines ... feeling so comfortable ... wonderful ... feeling so good all over and all the way through ... interesting to experience how you are ... at one and the same time ... aware that you are so relaxed and yet hardly aware of your body at all ... just a comfortable feeling of internal well-being.

Reduce bloating and distension

This script intentionally makes use of a variety of metaphors to appeal to different personalities. However, if you think it would be more appropriate, you could select only one metaphor and expand it to suit the individual. You need to consider the possibility that your client may pass wind during this relaxation and, if so, it is crucial to reduce any possible embarrassment by simply remarking 'that's it' 'that's right, letting it go now' or similar phrases.

Hypnosis makes use of so many amazing capabilities of the creative mind ... particularly for example the power of a thought to influence the body ... and also the power to make associations between one idea and another ... if you suggest a word or phrase to a person and allow them a few minutes to let their minds drift off into the realms of the unconscious and create associations ... it is fascinating to discover where they go in their minds and just what they come up with ... moving seamlessly *from one situation to another* ... *changing one attitude for another without questioning* that it can be done ... we are not bound by the limitations of the conscious mind that raises this or that objection ... defensive or fearful of change ... in free association we are open and creative and can *find inventive solutions* to all manner of problems ... emotional and physical.

> **Seeds the idea that the mind is creative in hypnosis and it can influence the body**

> **The unconscious mind seeks and find solutions without the limitations of the conscious mind**

And I tried this once ... I suggested the words 'ease bloating' to someone ... and this is where they went first in their imagination ... quite a commonplace scene where you are cycling along and realise that you have overfilled your tyres as the ride is too hard ... and you *need very gently to adjust the pressure* and *let some air out just very gently* to let it down until it is softer to allow a more comfortable ride.

> **Intentional change of pronoun to 'you'**

And then (they) drifted on to another kind of commonplace situation ... where you notice that the radiator is not functioning as well as it should because there is an airlock ... so you need to *find the key to release the air* and everyone who's ever

> **Omit this section if, in your country, it is not customary to use water filled radiators**

117

done this knows the trick is to *stay calm and to do it slowly and gently* ... so you release the air and not the water and when it's done the water fills up and replaces the released air so that the radiator *functions perfectly again* and the warmth spreads around the room.

And then drift to a more playful thought ... remembering what fun you can have as a child ... how the most simple things can please so much ... like playing with blowing bubbles or with brightly coloured balloons ... and of course in your imagination you can even play the game of ... *becoming the balloon and floating around the* room ... which is OK for a while and then you begin to *feel just how nice it would be to relax and have a good rest from floating ... reduce that (dis)tension ... let go of all the tension* and just *feel yourself gently deflating in the very nicest possible way ... simply loosen up the knot a little and let down the balloon gently ... gently ... relax all the tension and enjoy that flatter sensation* ... that balloon *becoming flatter and flatter* as ... you ... very calmly ... very slowly and comfortably ... *relax all the muscles and regain the feeling and the appearance of a very flat and very flexible balloon.*

And drifting from balloons to preparing a meal ... so easily done in free association ... where you are poaching something in a pan on the cooker and you need to be very careful to watch it and keep it very gently at a steady, low temperature ... not even letting it simmer ... keep an eye on it and watch for any signs that you need to reduce the temperature ... sometimes adjusting the lid to let out a little steam when you need to ... catch it in time so it can never boil over ... notice the signals to calm down the heat and do whatever you need to do ... make any necessary adjustments. And of course you need to keep an eye on the other pans and dishes too ... being careful not to have too many things on the go all at the same time ... leaving yourself adequate time to devote attention appropriately to all parts of the meal

Intentional moving away from 'somebody else's' free association to the client's own

People commonly describe the feeling of bloating in the abdomen as being like a balloon, tight and swollen

This is a metaphor about watching for signs of pressure which cause tension and taking action to pre-empt it or to reduce it before it's too late. In the pre-induction talk it would be useful to discuss such signs and signals

... adjusting ... reducing ... taking time to relax and enjoy the tasting ... not trying to do too many things at the same time.

And you ... of course ... can find your own associations as you continue to rest here for a while ... wondering at the conscious or unconscious level which things you will cut down or cut out altogether to reduce the pressure in your life ... and reduce the pressure in your tummy/stomach/belly/abdomen ... which ways you will remind yourself to always take the time out to sit down while you eat ... eat much more slowly ... to chew your food very thoroughly ... to eat only small portions at one time ... give yourself some relaxing time to digest your food.

And just for a few more minutes you can *enjoy relaxing all the muscles even more than before* as you let your mind have free rein to drift where you will ... maybe finding some thought-provoking ideas ... maybe letting all the pressure out of your tyre ... or your radiator ... your balloon ... or adjusting the controls as you cook ... adjusting the pan lids ... or simply let all the excess air out with your breathing ... breathe it all away with each out breath.

You could go to the script *Relaxation of the digestive tract* coupled with letting go of any stress with the out breath. You can also choose to intersperse words and phrases such as: *subsiding now ... pressure reducing ... gently loosening any knots ... letting go of any possible remaining tension ... flattening out ... wonderfully flat ... gently ... functioning perfectly.* **Or you may prefer to go immediately to a suitable trance reorientation**

Soothing liquid calm

Use the *Mental massage* script or any other gentle relaxing induction.

And all of the time you've been relaxing your body ... your mind has been becoming more and more creative so that now it can seem completely natural to use your mind to *soothe your body on the inside* ... so let yourself do that now ... I wonder where you would store the most precious soothing liquid designed to calm your whole digestive system? In a cupboard? ... On a shelf? ... Wherever it is ... go there now and find the bottle of liquid calm for your stomach ... liquid calm for your intestines ... I wonder what colour it is ... take the bottle in your hand and give it a shake ... find a spoon ... take a spoonful ... mmm ... it tastes so pleasant ... and has the most calming effect ... and as it slips down your throat ... into the oesophagus ... (that passageway that leads down into the stomach) ... feel the liquid soothing and calming all the way down ... calming any possible inflamed areas ... coating the linings with a protective, soothing balm ... easing everything along its path and into the stomach ... that's it ... now take another spoonful of calm and become aware of how all the nerves are calm and comfortable ... all the muscles of your digestive tract are working gently and firmly ... yet unobtrusively ... with a regular rhythmic, rippling movement ... all the parts of the digestive system working together in a calm and co-ordinated way ... moving the food matter along ... you feel so calm and relaxed ... the muscles contracting gently yet firmly just as they should ... the nerves calmly transmitting information from one place to the next so that everything functions perfectly to ensure steady, calm progress ... not too fast and not too slow ... this amazing liquid aids the digestion of food in the stomach so the whole process happens just as It should ... just as it's supposed to ... and it's fine to *trust your body to do all of this for you easily and effortlessly* ... as the soothing liquid continues to ease the process

This is a simplified fantasy visualisation of the whole digestive process

Visual

Gustatory

Kinaesthetic

Use your most soothing and calming voice tone to increase the effect

'unobtrusively' **is a useful word since generally people with IBS tend to be more sensitive to internal sensations than those without IBS symptoms**

of digestion … moving the partially digested food all the way down from the stomach into the small intestine … working with all the digestive enzymes (from the pancreas and the liver) … to extract all the nutrients and everything needed for the body's well-being and perfect functioning … and transport them around the body … all the digestive processes working perfectly … then the wonderful soothing liquid eases the passage of the remaining waste matter into the large intestine for the next stage of the process … the whole process is calm and easy … and … now this waste matter is moved along on its controlled journey towards its eventual exit … which will be calm and comfortable at the time and place of your choosing … everything is moving at just the right speed … not too fast … not too slow … just the right consistency … all being gathered and moved along gently and firmly … the liquid balm reducing any gases and easing and controlling the journey till it reaches the storage place in the colon … where it will rest comfortably until it is passed out of your body at a time and place of your choosing … you are completely in control … it's passed comfortably and fully … complete evacuation of all the waste matter … any possible, remaining gas passed gently … leaving you feeling so comfortable and pleasantly empty … that you can *forget all about the procedure at the conscious level*, allowing your unconscious mind to do all the remembering it needs … while your conscious mind can *enjoy thinking about something else entirely* … your body remains calm and comfortable … nothing disturbing it all … it's so calm and comfortable that *you're hardly aware of your body at all* as you just *get on with your life in the way that you want.*

Every night when you go to bed take a couple of minutes as you are relaxing and winding down from your day … to imagine your bottle of soothing, calming liquid (what colour was it?) and take a couple of spoonfuls … running through the procedure just as we've done here today … and every time you do

Regular practice reinforces the calming effect of the visualisation. Set this for homework

this, your body is reinforcing its new learning so that each day it will seem more and more natural that you feel comfortable and at ease.

And if ever during the daytime, you were to want a little extra calm and comfort in your stomach/ abdomen/belly/tummy ... just take time out for a moment to ... stop and close your eyes ... reach for that liquid calm ... take a spoonful ... and notice how all the internal muscles begin to relax ... and the tiny little nerve endings start to calm down ... your whole system is calming down ... that's right.

In addition to night-time practice, a quick visualisation can be used as a trigger for calm as and when required. However, the use of the wording, 'if ever during the daytime, you were to want' suggests that this need might not arise very often!

Take a moment or two just before we draw this session to a close ... to get a sense of how things are going to be ... now that you have found a way to calm your whole digestive system ... see yourself in your mind's eye ... looking more calm and confident as you go through your daily life ... at work ... at home ... *looking and feeling comfortable* and even your voice *sounding* more relaxed than before ... notice how *you are altogether more outwardly focused* ... appreciate how *you are spending far more time simply enjoying yourself* ... doing whatever you want to do ... hardly aware of your body at all ... forgetting to remember or remembering to *forget about your body* and simply enjoying being you ... well done.

'Future pace' the client's desired outcome of a calmer digestive process. Enrich the visualisation with details of their everyday life

VAK

Go to a suitable trance reorientation

The river

A metaphorical journey through the entire digestive process including optional sections which deal with constipation and diarrhoea. It is very helpful to teach self-hypnosis and have them regularly visualise simplified versions of this at home. This both reinforces their response and gives a tool to use during bouts of IBS.

And you can choose which way you decide to imagine taking a rather unusual journey into your inner self ... in fact ... a journey into all the passageways of your digestive system ... you may *see everything very clearly* just as though you are looking at a movie ... or you may just *get a sense of being there on this interesting journey* ... you could imagine first taking a couple of sips of water and just slipping down your throat and into the oesophagus where ... quite amazingly ... you will find yourself on the bank of a river where there is a small motorboat moored at a landing stage ... just waiting for you to step into it ... *make yourself very comfortable* and you can begin your journey down the river ... take your place at the helm on this journey of discovery and check out *all the controls* ... some you will recognise ... like the speed controls and some of the others may be quite new to you ... the important thing is that you will find that *you have all the controls that you need.*

'get a sense of' **makes it easy for people who are less visual in their imagination**

The use of 'quite amazingly' **pre-empts possible disbelief or unwillingness to accept the metaphor of the digestive system as a river**

And as you move along down the river you can become aware of how that river feels today ... whether it's smooth ... or if it is a little bit choppy ... and notice now, if you will, that one of the controls is a 'water calmer' (I told you that some of the controls were rather unusual) ... so whenever you find that the water is at all choppy ... all you need to do is place your hand on the calming control ... that's it ... try it out right now ... take your hand and place it there now ... and ... become aware of a gentle spread of calm and comfort ... notice how it automatically calms that choppiness so the river flows smoothly and gently along ... that's it ... so you can safely remove your hand from the control whenever

An option here would be to direct them to put their hand on their tummy if you can do it without disturbing the flow of the metaphor

you want to ... knowing that you can turn it on again any time you need to do so.

And as you continue your journey ... before long you may notice that there is a sign warning you that you will soon be approaching the stomach rapids ... where, of course, it is perfectly normal for the water to become a little more choppy ... and right there on the control panel you will find a special lever, which will *automatically control the smoothness of the flow*... reach out and touch that lever now and notice how everything around you is calming down ... flowing at just the right pace and in just the right way for comfort and ease ... so that you can continue to feel in control as you steer through the waters that are beginning to be less choppy now ... *everything moving* steadily *along as you relax and enjoy the trip*.

Good ... the river is flowing really smoothly and calmly again now ... *you are completely in control* here and you can continue along the journey into the small intestine ... you will find that the river is flowing along really well and you are enjoying your trip along all the twists and turns of this stretch of water ... *moving along calmly and steadily* ...*the river flowing along really smoothly and easily* ... but take care ... because up ahead there's an area where the reeds grow thickly and very strongly and from time to time they can get caught up in the propellers ... so steer carefully to avoid them if you can ... but *stay cool/ calm* because you know you've got your boat hook on board if you should need it ... *you know what to do and how to do it* ... If at any time ... you were to notice that kind of griping or cramping sensation low down in the boat ... it just means that the reeds are getting tangled up and dragging on the propeller blades ... so you *slow right down ... stay very calm now ... stretch out* the boat hook ... and just *ease* the reed out ... yes ... ease it out of the blades ... *very, very gently yet firmly ... just unwind* the blades and *ease it out* ... and you will notice that it's already

124

beginning to *free itself* … yes … that's it … easy does it … *you know just how to do it … slow down … take it easy … take your time* … and … good … now it's free … and you can *feel how good it is* to cruise along again … a nice clear stretch of water now … moving along nicely … the current is quite strong here and *moving along any sludge that's collected on the river bed … everything moving along nicely* … that's it.

And … as the journey continues … from time to time there are some stretches of the river where you need to be on the lookout for some boulders along the river bed where … in the past … some of the sludge has had a tendency to get a bit caught up … the current is a bit weak here so you might have to help out … look down into the water … does it look really murky and muddy? … If so, it could be that you need to use your 'dredge control' to dredge up any old rubbish/garbage or stones that have collected over time and then *the current can take over and drag it along … take as long as you need* … some people even find that there is some emotional baggage … stresses or strains … down there at the bottom of the river that has got(ten) caught up in the reeds … just *place your hand on the control and let your unconscious mind do everything that needs to be done to free it and move it along … take all the time you need* … and what's really special is that your unconscious mind already knows how to do this for you without any conscious effort on your part at all … and when you're done … (let me know) you can take your hand off the control and you will find that the river is flowing along really well … and you are enjoying your trip along all the twists and turns of this stretch of water … moving along calmly and steadily … steadily and calmly.

Give more time or a little more direction here if your pre-trance discussion indicates emotional causes of withholding

Leave plenty of time for this to be carried out. You can check in with them to see if they need more time or more help

Use this section if the patient suffers from diarrhoea. Go to the following section if they suffer from constipation. Sometimes they suffer from both conditions intermittently, in which case you can include both sections

And as you continue your journey … you come to a different stretch of river known as the large intestine … and sometimes the waters can get a bit high and fast here … and the riverbanks can even need to be shored up a bit … how useful that … not only do *you have all the controls* at your fingertips to *slow yourself right down* … but you also have a team of helpers who are there on hand on the riverbank ready and waiting to assist you … there is a storehouse with all the equipment you need … and *all the resources you need* too … you might even want to get your team to help you shut the floodgates in the dam … the gates are operated with calm and patience … take some time to do that now … if you need some extra calm and patience, it's good to know *you've plenty of it in the storehouse* … and if you also need to shore up the banks with strong belief in yourself … it's a relief to know that *self-belief is also there in abundance* … just look into your storehouse and you will find plenty of evidence that *you are stronger than you thought* … you can *handle things calmly and competently* … and one of the best resources in your store is an ability to *be a good learner* … great … each time you sail down your river you *become more and more adept* at negotiating your way through … more and more skilled at slowing things down whenever you need to … *more and more skilled at shutting the floodgates quickly and firmly.*

Use this section if the patient suffers from constipation

And as you continue your journey you come to a different stretch of river known as the large intestine where sometimes the current is a bit weak and a bit slow … sometimes the sludge is a bit reluctant to move along … and the water gets very murky indeed … the level of the water is very low … the river can get a bit sluggish … even be in danger of running dry when there is too little rain … (of course

Optional Diarrhoea Section

You could elaborate on the 'team of helpers' **as appropriate, using for example 'the strong part of you' or 'the practical part of you' or 'the patient part of you'**

Include the client's relevant abilities and emotional resources that you have elicited in your pre-induction talk

Reassuring to hear that you improve as you learn and practise

Optional Constipation Section

in a similar way ... you need to *drink enough water* ... *eat a good diet* ... for your system to function at its best) ... but here in your boat it's the time when you need to press the dredger control once again and *move things along* ... that's it ... *drag the sludge along the river bed* ... and place your hand on the speed control and *hasten things along* ... you *handle things calmly and competently* ... and isn't it useful to know that there is a store cupboard in the boat full of helpful resources ... why don't you open it up and see what's there? ... As soon as you open it, optimism comes tumbling out and as you pick it up in your hands, it spreads all through you ... a positive bright feeling that lets you know *everything will be fine* ... have a look inside and see what else is there ... you can *find just what you need* ... yes ... great ... and *do please find one of the best resources in your entire store* ... that's right ... it's the ability to *be a good learner* ... so that each time you sail down your river, you *become more and more adept* at negotiating your way through ... *more and more skilled* at knowing where and when to *speed things up whenever you need to* ... *be more and more active* in your approach ... well done.

You can also search around in the store for a bit more ability to *focus outwardly* ... you might also want to offload some tension ... offload a bit of *over*sensitivity ... that's fine ... take a moment or two to do that so that you find you can *take things more easily* ... *take things in your stride* ... become less *overly* aware of physical sensation ... become less *overly* aware of emotional sensibilities ... and ... as you do, you will find that *the river journey becomes more pleasant and easy every day* ... *everything moving along steadily, easily, at just the right speed for you* ... you can *speed up or slow down just as you want to* ... until *you regularly arrive at the draw-bridge just before the river opens out into the sea* ... sometimes you need to *wait your turn* till the draw-bridge lifts up which you *do patiently and easily* but mostly now *the river journey has become so easy*

Drinking sufficient fluid is very important
Don't become involved in specifics of diet. Some medical opinion now questions the advisability of inclusion of too much fibre and vegetable in the diet for certain cases of IBS

Allow plenty of pauses for them to find the resources they need

Activity is important in relieving a sluggish elimination system

People with IBS are often overly focused on inner sensations

Emphasize 'over' **in the word** '*over*sensitivity'

'Emphasize the word 'overly' **in** '*overly* aware'

Emphasize the word 'regularly'

and natural that you *arrive at the drawbridge at just the right time* ... time for you to have your breakfast or evening meal before the bridge lifts up and the boat can easily sail through ... you *feel so comfortable and so at ease* that life on the river becomes second nature to you ... and I don't know exactly *how* soon it will be ... but I do *know it will be very soon* ... that it becomes almost difficult to remember the journey as it once was ... so easy to forget and much easier to *remember that a journey down the river is just plain sailing now* ... and you can *enjoy sailing out to sea every day.*

A common time for a bowel movement is immediately following a main meal

Emphasize the word 'how' in 'I don't know exactly *how* soon'

Go to a suitable trance reorientation

Variations, Adaptations and Recommendations

This metaphor could be simplified by losing much of the detail and merely asking the patient to imagine the digestive system as a river. You could invite them to imagine the water flowing more quickly or more slowly as appropriate, and have currents moving the sludge along the river bed as relevant to the individual.

Urinary Incontinence and Bladder Retraining

Considerations

Urinary frequency refers to an increased need to pass urine at frequent intervals. It is important to differentiate between an increase in urine production, as in diabetes incipidus, and a need to pass small amounts of urine at frequent intervals. The latter occurs in bladder infections, stones, bladder tumour, or obstruction, as in prostatic enlargement for example.

Only treat patients after medical diagnosis and with agreement of a medical practitioner. It is essential to have problems medically investigated, diagnosed and appropriately treated. Where bladder retraining has been advised, hypnotherapy can be very helpful.

How can hypnotherapy help?

- Maintain motivation to carry out the exercise plan as directed by the physician.
- Maintain motivation to drink appropriately.
- Lower anxiety. Anxiety in itself can also be a cause of frequency and urge problems, and work as a self-fulfilling prophecy.
- Create a positive mindset and deal with setbacks.
- Intensify positive beliefs and increase patience.
- Overcome embarrassment.
- Speed up progress and congratulate self on progress achieved.
- Set anchors for control and resistance to triggers.

Overcome daytime frequency

Frequency refers to feeling the need to pass urine at very or 'over' frequent intervals even when the bladder has good physical capacity. 'Normal' frequency will vary from person to person, with age, with the amount of fluid intake and with the intake of irritants to the bladder, for example coffee, tea, cola and alcohol. It is possible to get into the habit of responding to the most minor of signals long before it is necessary 'just to be on the safe side'. However, three to four hourly intervals between needing to pass urine is generally considered 'normal'.

Overcome urgency

Urge incontinence is the development of an overpowering need to pass urine NOW. It may not necessarily be linked to frequency, although it often is. Urgency can be associated with a leakage of urine ranging from a few drops to a complete soaking. The cause is often purely psychological as investigations do not reveal any abnormality in any part of the urinary system or urinary bladder thus it is well treated with hypnosis.

The feeling of urgency can be precipitated by various factors, some of which include:

- Running water
- Washing of hands
- Being in the cold
- Arriving home
- Approaching/opening the bathroom door
- Merely the thought of needing to go
- Memory of a previous lack of control.

Variations, Adaptations and Recommendations

In addition to the two scripts given here, extracts from certain scripts in the following sections will be found useful:

- *Dissociation of parts* could be useful, as could several other extracts in the *Coping with Pain* section. An adaptation of the *Recovery from surgery* script would also be suitable. Where there is significant anxiety, the section *Anxiety, Panic, Phobias*, notably *Desensitisation* and *Travel toilet phobia* could provide useful material to draw on.

- Discuss with your client a hierarchy of 'accident situations' and combine this with setting sensible goals with small steps at first for gradually increasing the time between visits to the toilet/lavatory/bathroom. Many clients suffer from lack of confidence and self-esteem because of the embarrassing nature of the problem and so will benefit from additional ego strengthening.

Bladder retraining to overcome daytime frequency, urgency and possible leakage

Be sure that your client has visited the bathroom before using the script. Use the words 'to make yourself comfortable' as you do not want to suggest the possibility of accident.

And feeling as pleasantly comfortable and relaxed as you do right now ... isn't it nice to know that this is the ideal state for you to be in as you learn to retrain your bladder ... our minds learn best when we are relaxed and focused and our bodies learn best when we are comfortable and at ease ... so do feel free to *increase your comfort* as you *relax even more deeply* as we go on.

It's comforting to be told that you are in the 'ideal state' **for learning**

Embedded commands

Now you already know that bladders can become overactive for a variety of reasons and ... you also know that bladders can be retrained to *respond more calmly and in a more controlled way.* Now, for whatever reason ... over time your bladder has learned to become **over**responsive to over enthusiastic signals ... now of course in one way this is good news since it tells us that *your bladder is good at learning* ... it's just that it has overdone it and it's time to *learn a different ... more appropriate way to respond* ... and as your bladder knows how to learn ... it can *enjoy learning more suitable responses* which will immensely improve the quality of your life.

Bladders can be retrained

Reframing the bladder as being 'good at learning' **gives a positive base to begin the retraining process**

You know from your medical history that your bladder has had a tendency to want to be emptied long before it's really full ... and because you also know that ... in reality ... it has plenty more capacity ... it needs to *learn to hold on a little longer before it empties* ... now as I said before ... you know all of that *consciously* but I would like you to take a moment now to mentally and silently explain to *your unconscious* mind ... that's the part of you responsible for all your body's autonomic processes such as controlling your bladder ... explain that your bladder has lots more capacity and can *hold on far longer*

The bladder is not full. The signals are faulty or overenthusiastic

than it used to do ... do that now and let me know when you've done so. [Pause] Excellent ... so your bladder now *understands* it can *hold on far longer than before* but it also needs to *get into the habit of holding on a bit longer ... and then a bit longer still ... and then even a bit longer than you ever dreamed you could ... couldn't you?*

And one of the best ways to learn a new habit is to use your conscious mind and your unconscious mind together ... *you can achieve outstanding results* ... so consciously now I want you to ... think about yourself at home in that situation/those situations where previously your bladder was being over-enthusiastic about wanting to empty itself ... let your unconscious mind ... the part of you that is good at imagining ... *form an image* of you in that situation/those situations ... or just get a very real sense of being there now ... remind yourself that your bladder has lots more room/much more capacity so that it's safe to *relax and ignore that faulty signal* and see that picture of you ... first noticing a faulty urge ... and then immediately reminding yourself that your bladder has plenty more capacity so you can stay calm ... remind yourself that you can hold on ... it's safe for you to *resist that mistaken urge ... squeeze your sphincter/pelvic floor muscles* ... and do something to distract yourself for a few minutes ... your unconscious mind can *take control, and safely ignore the urge* as you become mentally engaged in something else ... well done.

Guide them through specific situations already placed in a hierarchy of difficulty or awkwardness or let them run through a selection in their own imagination

Include several repetitions of the suggestions to resist the urge and successfully distract themselves

I want you to know that throughout this period of training your unconscious mind will be sifting through all the internal resources you need ... so there will be no need to consciously try to *be patient with yourself as you regularly train and practise this new skill* ... your unconscious mind will ensure you *find all the patience and resilience you need* ... so it will *feel perfectly natural* that *you remain determined to carry out all these strengthening exercises every-day ... you remain very patient ... when you pass*

A series of embedded commands

Motivation to keep up the physical practice of the prescribed exercises

urine you can practise stopping and starting the flow at will ... and you find yourself focusing on your progress ... congratulating yourself on each little positive step along the way ... you *notice yourself seeing all kinds of aspects of your life in a positive light ...* not only about your progress with your bladder training but in all areas of your everyday life ... you are more confident and you enjoy how optimistic you are ... and I wonder whether you will find yourself being surprised by the fact that the old embarrassment slipped away so easily or whether it will be difficult to remember ... and ... after all ... why should you? ... that it was ever there at all.

Presupposition that progress with bladder retraining has already occurred

And I'm wondering ... although I'm sure *you're very certain* ... which aspects of your life will be improved *first* as you *gain more confidence and control of your bladder* ... and which aspect gives you most satisfaction? Will it be that you can *feel more relaxed* when you are out and about? ... Or when you're at work? ... Or at home? ... Or with other people? ... Or will it be that you *feel more confident that you can hold on for the right time and the right place*? ... Or will it be that after a while things will have improved so much that you won't even have to think about it at all? ... Won't even have to think about it at all as *you will have complete control of your bladder at both the conscious and unconscious level.*

'which aspects of your life will be improved first' **presupposes there will be improvement in several aspects**

Recommended reorientation: *Unconscious continuation.* (However, you might like to omit or reword the suggestion about noticing other people's responses)

Bladder retraining to overcome urge incontinence

This is an adaptation of the previous script. The first two and the last two sections are the same but the middle sections are different and deal specifically with resisting the urge and responding only to a given signal.

Read the middle sections before your pre-trance discussion.

Be sure that your client has visited the bathroom before using the script. Use the words 'to make yourself comfortable' as you do not want to suggest the possibility of accident.

And feeling as pleasantly comfortable and relaxed as you do right now ... isn't it nice to know that this is the ideal state for you to be in as you learn to retrain your bladder ... our minds learn best when we are relaxed and focused and our bodies learn best when we are comfortable and at ease ... so do feel free to *increase your comfort* as you *relax even more deeply* as we go on.

It's comforting to be told that you are in the 'ideal state' **for learning**

Embedded commands

Now you already know that bladders can become overactive for a variety of reasons and you also know that bladders can be retrained to *respond more calmly and in a more controlled way.* For whatever reason over time your bladder has learned to become **over**responsive to signals ... now of course in one way this is good news since it tells us that your bladder is good at learning ... it's just that it has overdone it and it's time to learn a different ... more appropriate way to respond ... and as your bladder knows how to learn ... it can enjoy learning more suitable responses which will immensely improve the quality of your life.

Bladders can be retrained

Reframing the bladder as being 'good at learning' **gives a positive base to begin the retraining process**

Now you know from your medical history that your bladder has had a tendency to respond to signals overenthusiastically and it needs to slow down ... stay calm ... *learn to hold on longer and only* respond when you give it the correct signal ... now as I said before ... you know all of that *consciously* but I would like you to take a moment now to mentally and silently explain to *your unconscious* mind ... that's the part of you responsible for all your body's autonomic processes such as controlling your bladder ... explain that your bladder has lots more capacity and can *hold on far longer than it used to do* ... it can *wait till you give it your chosen signal* ... do that now and let me know when you've done so. [Pause] Excellent ... so your bladder now **understands** it can *hold on far longer than before* ... and it also needs to **get into the habit** of holding on a bit longer ... and a bit longer still ... every day and every night your ability to *be in control of that urge* becomes a bit stronger and a bit stronger still.

And one of the best ways to learn a new habit is to use your conscious mind and your unconscious mind together ... *you can achieve outstanding results* ... so consciously now I want you to think about yourself ... and see yourself just as you described to me ... walking up to your front door ... getting your door key in your hand ... (where *previously* your bladder used to get overenthusiastic about wanting to empty itself) ... let your unconscious mind ... the part of you that is good at imagining ... form an image of yourself in that situation now ... or just get a very real sense of being there now ... remind yourself that *you are in control of your bladder* ... completely in control ... *you will only start the flow at the time and place of your choosing* ... and see that picture of you ... reminding yourself that your bladder has plenty more capacity so you can stay calm ... remind yourself that you can hold on ... it's safe for you to resist that premature urge ... *squeeze your sphincter/pelvic floor muscles* as if you were already stopping the flow ... that's right, squeezing your muscles with superb control ... and think about something else ... preparing the dinner/ watching your favourite film/that wonderfully calm image we spoke about ... your unconscious mind

Agree with the client beforehand a mental signal for starting the flow, e.g. 'Let's go now'/'Start the flow'

Go through a detailed guided visualisation of resisting each of the 'urge triggers' experienced by your patient

Running water, washing of hands, being in the cold, putting the key in the front door, opening the toilet/bathroom door are frequently experienced triggers for starting the flow too soon. Indeed even *the thought* that they may need to go soon can act as trigger for some people

can *take control and safely resist the urge* as you enjoy thinking about something else entirely ... you know *you are in charge of your bladder* now ... see yourself calmly <u>putting the key in the door ... walking in calmly and deliberately</u> ... walking steadily to the bathroom/toilet/lavatory ... you can hold on easily and strongly ... take your time to adjust your clothes as appropriate ... you know you have plenty of time and you stay in control ... and only when the time is right for you ...you will respond to the signal ... as soon as you <u>take aim/sit on the seat/you hover over the seat/you are ready to go</u> ... and only when *you* decide ... you give yourself the mental signal, '<u>Let's go now'/'Start the flow'</u> and you can begin. ... Perfectly done.

Be explicit. The mind and the body want clear signals. Talk through implications of signals beforehand. It is not always appropriate, for example, to sit on an unclean lavatory seat!

I want you to know that throughout this period of retraining ... your unconscious mind will be sifting through all the internal resources you need ... so there will be no need to consciously try to *be patient with yourself as you regularly train and practise this new skill* ... your unconscious mind will ensure you *find all the calm, the patience and resilience you need* ... so it will *feel perfectly natural* that *you remain determined to carry out all these strengthening exercises every day ... when you pass urine you can practise stopping and starting the flow at will ... you remain very patient and you find yourself focusing on your progress* ... congratulating yourself on each little positive step along the way ... you *notice yourself seeing all kinds of different aspects of your life in a positive light* ... not only about your progress with your bladder training but in all areas of your everyday life ... you are more confident and you enjoy how very optimistic you are feeling these days ... and I wonder whether you will find yourself being surprised by the fact that the old embarrassment slipped away so easily or whether it will be difficult to remember ... and ... after all ... why should you? ... that it was ever there at all.

A series of embedded commands

Motivation to keep up the physical practice of the prescribed exercises

Presupposition that progress with bladder retraining has already occurred

And I'm wondering … but I'm sure you are very certain … which aspects of your life will be improved first as you *gain more confidence and control of your bladder* … and which aspect gives you most satisfaction? Will it be that you can *feel more relaxed* when you are out and about? … Or when you're at work? … Or at home? … Or with other people? … Or will it be that you *feel more confident that you can hold on for the right time and the right place*? … Or will it be that after a while things will have improved so much that you won't even have to think about it at all? … Won't even have to think about it at all as you will have complete control of your bladder at both the conscious and unconscious level.

'which aspects of your life will be improved first' **presupposes there will be improvement in several aspects**

Recommended reorientation: *Unconscious continuation.* (However, you might like to omit or reword the suggestion about noticing other people's responses)

Surgery: Preparation and Recovery

Preparation for surgery

You've told me that you are going to have an operation/procedure and that you'd like me to help you approach this in a way that is calm and comfortable and the wonderful thing about hypnosis is that in this special state ... not only will your mind be calm and at ease but your body too can *be comfortable, at ease and prepared for every step of the way.*

Shows you have been listening and identifies objectives. Include the client's own words

Maybe you already know that when a person is physically very comfortable and calm and deeply relaxed ... their mind can *take on board positive suggestions* that will help them *achieve whatever it is that they want to achieve.*

Introduces the idea of the mind accepting positive suggestions and, at the same time, giving an embedded command to take on positive suggestions and achieve their aims

So the first thing to do is for me to help you *become pleasantly relaxed ... feel very comfortable* and *let your mind drift off* to a place in your imagination where you feel very much at ease, maybe even feel a bit drowsy while you listen. Make it some pleasant, calming place where you can *feel very, very comfortable ... comfortable in yourself* ... comfortable about yourself in every way ... maybe in some special calming garden ... or maybe on a beach somewhere ... or maybe just in some calm place in you ... wherever you are ... just allow all the muscles in your body to *let go and relax ...* and ... (how good is that?) ... to *feel that comfort and ease* as you settle into this safe daydreamy state ... I think we all like to *dream and feel safe* and *feel comfortable* as we *take some time to relax* ... and it's so pleasant here that it's very comforting to know that you can float into this place whenever you want to have some peace and quiet ... let the doctors get on with their healing work for example ... while you *take some time out to enjoy a pleasant and peaceful daydream.*

Allows the patient to select their own calming place

Keeping the voice light and questioning in tone

A truism which encourages mental agreement

And now I'm going to show you how *you* yourself can *develop your level of relaxation a little more* and

138

then a little more still ... so you are able to *enjoy a very comfortable level of relaxation* now as you *listen to the calming and positive suggestions* that you need to prepare your mind and body ... and later too ... *when*ever and *where*ver you want to increase your calm and relaxation. ... your own mind can control the degree of relaxation you achieve ... just say to yourself, really meaning it ... 'with each in breath I am breathing in calm and comfort ... and with each out breath I am breathing out any possible tension and all the muscles in my body are relaxing' [Pause] and then notice how your body follows your thought and begins to *feel more and more comfortable ... more and more deeply relaxed and calm ...* might even feel heavier and heavier ... that's right ... *all the way through* ... isn't that interesting how your own mind can direct your body?

> Introduces the idea of the patient being in control of the relaxation, both now and in the future too

> Seeds the idea of the mind directing the body

The more you practise it, the more skilled you become ... [Pause] that's right ... all the muscles relaxing ... and you can *continue doing this* throughout your whole body ... your feet ... *relaxed and calm* ... your legs ... *relaxed and calm* ... the trunk of your body ... *relaxed and calm* ... your chest ... *relaxed and calm* ... your hands ... *relaxed and calm* ... your arms ... *relaxed and calm* ... your shoulders ... *relaxed and calm* ... your neck ... *relaxed and calm* ... your head ... *relaxed and calm* as you continue following my voice ... until your whole body has become so comfortable ... and ... at the same time ... in a rather unusual and pleasant way ... you can be hardly aware of your body at all ... just aware of a sense of comfort all the way through ... that's right. [Pause]

> You can elaborate on this relaxation if you want to do so, by repeating the instruction above about 'in and out breaths' with each part of the body you mention. Allow a sufficient pause for the patient to repeat the words to themselves and to allow the responses to occur

And each time you do this on your own ... *any* time ... *any* place ... you will *become more deeply relaxed, more easily and more swiftly than before ... and you know you can even increase those wonderful feelings of relaxation by using the words calm and relax* ... that's right ... *calm and relax* ... you can let

> Presupposes they will practise this on their own outside the treatment session

139

them spread over you now as I say those words now ... *calm and relax* ... that's it.

And now in this comfortable state of relaxation ... which you can notice will *become even deeper with each out breath* ... and ... as it does ... your own mind is creating this special state of hypnosis where you can become more aware of the part that your unconscious mind plays in regulating all the processes of your physical body ... your breathing ... the beating of your heart ... your kidneys cleansing your system ... your skin cells renewing ... your whole digestive system ... all of this happening outside of your normal everyday awareness ... but in this heightened hypnotic state of awareness there can also be heightened communication between the conscious and the unconscious parts of your mind and body ... and in an unusual kind of a way ... this process can just be achieved with your breathing.

Introduces the idea of the hypnotic state heightening conscious–unconscious communication

Stating that something can happen 'in an unusual kind of a way' **allows the acceptance of a rather unusual idea**

So I'm going to suggest words to communicate with your breathing ... simply breathe these words ... (or turn them into your own words) ... into your unconscious awareness ... and your unconscious mind will understand completely ... it will then communicate this to your body in its own wonderful, mysterious way so that *every cell and every atom of your body will be calm and prepared* for every detail of the procedure ... you see ... your brain produces calming neurotransmitters which can *fill your mind and body with calm* ... that's right *calm and relax your mind and body* ... you can *let calm spread through you right now* as I say these words ... *calm and relax*.

Omit the idea of breathing if you prefer, and simply ask them to have a mental conversation (but I have found that people respond well to the idea of breathing the words)

The words '*calm and relax*' **become an auditory anchor and are repeated throughout the section**

So now please take a good deep breath and just breathe these words into your unconscious so they will be communicated to your body ... 'you are soon going to have *an operation/some treatment which*

140

is specifically to help you get well/better as soon as possible'. [Pause] That's it ... your body now *understands this operation/treatment is to enhance your health and well-being* ... so all the systems of your body can *be well prepared ... no surprises ... just calm and relaxed.*

Take another deep breath and breathe this message into your skin ... 'Because you know that everything is designed to help you get well in the best possible way for you ... you can welcome the surgeon's incision/intervention ... *your skin and every cell of your body will be prepared and agreeable to this incision* knowing that it allows the surgeon to make any necessary repairs ... allows them to remove any parts necessary for your overall good and healing.' [Pause] That's it ... *your mind and body are prepared and calm and relaxed.*

With your breathing ... explain to every internal organ that *'any manipulation or repair is for your overall good and well-being'* ... explain that *'every internal organ can stay calm and flexible so every procedure can be welcomed'*. That's it ... simply breathe the words into your body. [Pause] That's it ... *your mind and body are prepared and calm and relaxed* ... your mind welcomes this ... your body welcomes this ... *calm and relax.*

So now every part of you understands that all of this treatment is in your very best interests ... you can trust your unconscious mind to regulate and adapt your blood flow in the most appropriate and helpful way, so that every aspect of you is in full co-operation with your surgeon/doctor/medical team ... just as later ... while you are recovering ... your unconscious mind will know how to continue to direct that flow of blood with all its healing nutrients ... to just the right part and in just the right way for excellent/easy/rapid healing ... all of this will happen at the unconscious level so there's no need for you to be consciously aware of it at all ... it's good that you can trust your unconscious mind to know just what to do.

Trust the unconscious mind

Take a moment now to breathe into your unconscious mind and body any positive personal message or request of your own. [Pause] That's good.

One more deep breath now as you *ask your mind to turn on its positive filter this very moment* so that before, during and after your operation you will *disregard any possible careless or tactless talk or words* that could possibly be misinterpreted in any way … such words have absolutely no importance to you … nothing will bother or disturb you … at *a deep inner level you will have a sense of peace and calm and security all over and all the way through* … so that now … and sooner and later … a sense of serenity will speed your recovery.

This suggestion is very important since friends, family and even medical staff can unintentionally cause anxiety or negativity through ill-thought-out remarks. There seems to be anecdotal evidence which suggests that patients even hear such remarks when fully or partially under anaesthetic

This sense of serenity will be there for you as you return to full conscious awareness once *the operation is successfully completed* … you can *be aware of a sense of calm and optimism when you wake* and *this calm, optimistic feeling will remain with you* as you are recovering … and as you are recovering your strength … all the natural healing forces of your body will be working for you … repairing … renewing … strengthening … your mind will *be thinking and feeling optimistically* … you will *find yourself coping well with any body* … *you will be coping positively with any effects of surgery* … *you will be coping with any situation* whether you are in a general ward or an individual room and … of course … once you are back at home again. There will be a sense of satisfaction that you have moved through the first stage and now your body's natural energy will be directed to the ongoing healing process.

Note the presupposition of *'the operation is successfully completed'*

This section includes lots of suggestions for positive, optimistic recovery

Separation of the words *any* **and** *body* **in the phrase** *'coping well with any body'* **provides intentional ambiguity**

So you have had some excellent conscious and unconscious communication here today and I'm curious to know when you will *notice the results in your level of inner calm* … will it be before or after you

142

notice the optimism and positivity in your thinking? …
And I'm also wondering who … apart from yourself
… will be noticing the outer serenity and positivity
that seems to shine out from within you … well, I'm
not exactly sure in **which order** *all these things will
occur* … only that you will be delighted to *notice that
they do occur* … so now is the time for you to begin
to *reorient to the room* gently and slowly … bringing with you all these positive optimistic ideas and
expectations in both your mind and your body.

Go to a suitable trance reorientation

Variations, Adaptations and Recommendations

Suggestions to allay anxiety about the stay in the hospital itself:

- You will feel calm and at ease on the way to the hospital/as you arrive at the hospital.
- You will feel comfortable whether you are wearing your own clothes or a hospital gown.
- You will feel a quiet confidence when speaking to any of the medical team and quite comfortable with asking any and all the questions you may have.
- You take any pre-med procedures in your stride.
- Time will seem to pass surprisingly quickly as you comfort-ably and patiently await your turn.
- You welcome the anaesthetic as you know it will be good to sleep and drift off to a pleasant daydream while the doctors carry out the operation safely and well.
- Later when you wake you will look and feel remarkably good and know you are well on the road to rapid recovery.
- When it is mealtime you will find that your appetite has returned and you eat well.
- You will sleep calmly and comfortably and any hustle and bustle of hospital life will sound reassuring.
- Time will pass quickly and soon it will be time for you to return home where you will continue to recover rapidly and well.

Additional scripts

Scripts from the *Coping with Pain* section may also be useful, as will the script *Time distortion* in the *Miscellaneous* section.

Recovery from surgery: bathe in a lake with special healing properties

Allowing yourself just to let the sound of my voice relax you ... calm and comfort you as you listen ... noticing yourself responding to the sound of the voice ... feeling your body relax as waves of comfort and ease relax your mind ... knowing that later when your mind drifts off ... as it will do ... just listening and relaxing ... deeper and deeper ... you will be drawn back to the *sound* of the voice while the *message* of the voice can be absorbed at a deeper inner level without the need for conscious attention or effort ... you, merely welcoming the opportunity to relax the body and enjoy the rest.

VAK

Conscious attention on the voice while the unconscious absorbs meaning

'Enjoy the rest' **(relaxation) and** 'enjoy the rest' **(remainder of the session)**

And as you feel the voice relaxing you ... deeper and deeper ... going deeper and deeper with each out breath ... you are becoming aware of how your body relishes these moments of calm and how it allows all its natural healing forces to come into play and enhance the process of recovery ... and at times like this it's good to remember that simple healing processes in the body are continually working for us outside our conscious awareness ... how, for example, with nothing more than a little time, your skin heals itself when scratched or grazed or cut ... all on its own with no special external process or medical attention ... I wonder how many times throughout your life your skin has just healed over without your even thinking about it ... it somehow knows just how to do it all on its own ... and I wonder how ... right now ... you can *enhance that process* by imagining ... in whatever way is right for you ... this healing process occurring ... maybe you can see it in your mind's eye as a gentle beam of light that soothes as it heals every place it is directed on your body ... maybe you are even becoming aware of this healing taking place as I speak, possibly with a sense of warmth or gentle tingling ... or is it perhaps even with a calming coolness ? ... Maybe you just get

'feel the voice relaxing you' **... a deliberate choice of words to merge listening with feeling**

Everybody has experienced this so it is easy to relate to and reinforces the idea that the body has a natural healing ability

Brings in all the senses

Covers all possibilities

a sense of it happening ... whichever way ... your body instinctively knows the stages of cleansing, repairing and renewing so you don't have to know *how* it does it ... only know that it *does* do it ... so you can allow it to happen automatically, naturally as you drift into a healing dream ... everybody knows how to dream ... we do it every night ... whether we remember it or not ... and as you drift off into your very own healing dream, it's good to know that your mind becomes more creative in this state ... can create the dream and can create the state of serenity ... that ideal state for healing to take place ... and whether you can *see a wonderful lake* in your dream as you hear me mention it or merely *get a sense of its being there* is not really important at all ... you may choose only to listen to my words as I tell you of a wonderful lake which is the colour of spearmint ... the lake is surrounded by mountains with snow still visible on the tops in summer ... yet the air is warm from the rays of the sun with just that hint of mountain freshness and as you look at the lake the sun glints on the water and the purity of the blue green colour of the water amazes ... yes ... those amazing colours come from the minerals that over years and years have flowed down into the lake from the crystal clear mountain streams ... and since ancient times people have bathed in the lake to absorb the healing properties of the water.

> The suggestion that the mind is more creative in hypnosis, allows acceptance of the creation of dreams and serene states

> Gives the freedom to experience the visualisation of the lake in any chosen modality

> VAK

> The minerals add to the sense of the healing properties of the lake

And you too can allow yourself to see/get a sense of/imagine this lake (or a lake of your own creation) that has a wonderful atmosphere of peace and purity ... have a look now and notice any colours you see around you ... above you ... below you ... breathing in the pure fresh air ... possibly noticing refreshing scents on the air? ...Take a deep breath and feel your lungs appreciating it ... not only your lungs but your whole body ... and as you breathe out, you're relaxing even more than before ... and with each in breath, sensing the purifying air circulating around your body ... cleansing your entire body on the inside ... with each out breath breathing away

> If they don't like the lake you describe, this gives them the opportunity to create one of their own choosing

> Olfactory sense

145

any possible impurities ... feeling yourself drawn to the lake to bathe in the safe, shallow water with all the healing minerals ... first dipping your toe into the water and discovering to your delight that the temperature is perfect for you ... feeling the sand beneath your feet ...and if you'd like to, you can sit down or lie back since the water is shallow ... and ... as well as having therapeutic properties ... it has salts which make it completely buoyant so it holds you very safely as your skin absorbs all the minerals it needs into the body to enrich the healing process ... as you rest here for a while can you notice how *you are beginning to get a sense of wellness* ... feel as if the natural buoyancy of the therapeutic water is seeming to spread into your whole being/your soul ... a sense of inner well-being so strong that it seems to emanate from the very core of you ... sensations of vitality ... an inner voice that is reassuring and inspiring ... as though ... perhaps ... joyful music is filling you with a sense of renewal ... and a knowledge that *healing is well underway* ... that *the processes of regeneration and renewal are unstoppable now* ... they will continue as you breathe ... in every waking moment ... and as you sleep ... a wonderful restorative sleep.

And as you step out of the lake, drying yourself in the warmth of the sun, you can look back and down into the water and see your reflection sparkling up at you ... looking healthy and well ... moving easily and fluidly ... that inner vitality and confidence shining through ... hearing the voices of your family and friends telling you how very well you look. ... As each day you are feeling stronger ... each day you have a greater sense of energy ... each day you are more aware of an inner sense of emotional well-being ... each night you are sleeping soundly ... each night your body is recovering as it rests ... repairing, regenerating and renewing ... each night you are dreaming of happy times ahead so that when you wake in the morning you will feel refreshed and find yourself looking forward to a good day ahead. Very

'safe and shallow' pre-empts fear of stepping into the water

More reassurance

VAK

Suggestion that the healing process will continue regardless of conscious awareness of it

'Future paces' evidence of health and well-being

Suggestion that recovery time will pass quickly

146

soon, as the days and the weeks have passed by so speedily … you will be looking back and congratu-lating yourself on your excellent recovery … and realising that you yourself have now become part of the evidence that suggests that a sense of positivity, inner happiness and optimism truly does speed up the recovery process … well done!

And in a few moments time … already feeling so much more positive and optimistic you will be drifting back into full alert conscious awareness … not only of your surroundings here with me … but also of a wonderful sense of confidence and well-being the moment you open your eyes.

Go to a more formal trance reorientation if appropriate

Coping with Pain

Elements of pain

One important function of pain is to alert the sufferer to the possible need for medical attention, therefore it is crucial that you do not help a patient ignore or become less aware of sensations that should be taken as a warning. Proposed hypnotherapy treatment for pain relief is best approved by a medical practitioner before treating a client in order to afford protection to both the patient and the therapist.

Pain has many elements in addition to the physical sensations themselves. Tension is certainly an aspect that increases the perception of pain. When patients can be helped to relax, they can often experience much less discomfort than previously, which is why relaxation inductions can often work very well. Conversely, initially the pain may be so intense that relaxing proves too difficult so, in this case, it may be better first to focus on and analyse the sensations, and then change the focus and distract before bringing in the concept of relaxation.

Sometimes it is necessary for patients to explore the origins of pain, look for causes or functions before being able to be free of it or at least tolerate it with more equanimity. They may need to be guided through a process where they understand that by letting go of a memory of previously experienced pain they will also lessen their current discomfort.

Expectation of severe pain will also doubtless have a strong negative effect so helping a client change their expectations can have a very beneficial outcome.

Very often pain will be affected by emotion too, for example fear, anxiety, anger, resentment, sadness, or grief. A person may be grieving for loss of health, career and lifestyle or indeed potential loss of life itself. Naturally this would impact severely on their perception of the pain and their ability to tolerate it.

Externalisation, dissociation, relaxation, time distortion, distraction, compartmentalisation and use of metaphor are all useful strategies in helping a patient gain pain relief. As usual, guided visualisation of a positive outcome plus ego strengthening is always valuable. Most of these strategies are employed in the group of scripts which follow. A script with time distortion utilisation may be found in the *Miscellaneous* section.

Variations, Adaptations and Recommendations

The following three metaphors were not originally intended as complete scripts in themselves, although many people who have used them say that they proved to be more than sufficient with the addition of a trance termination. Rather, they are intended to be included within other scripts, or used as inductions/deepeners, or used as frameworks to which you can add direct suggestions and guided visualisations appropriate to the individual client. *Ease away knots of pain and tension*, which has good kinaesthetic appeal, could be added very successfully to either of the first two metaphors. Both the scripts in the *Surgery* section could also be easily and very usefully adapted and used in helping offer relief from pain.

Breathe out the colour of pain

Using the visual sense to imagine pain as a colour can help in the process of dissociation from painful physical sensations.

As you sit/lie there beginning to relax just a little more ... you can let yourself become aware of the surface beneath you ... supporting you ... holding you ... maybe you have cushions or pillows behind or beside you ... and if not there in reality ... maybe you can allow your creative mind to conjure up some cushions ... cushions full of calm ... full of comfort ... imagining you can feel the texture of these cushions ... feel the buoyancy of them ... seemingly *experiencing the mind and body as floating on cushions of calm and comfort ... feeling both the softness and yet the amazing support of the cushions ... absorbing uplifting feelings from the cushions ...* everything positive they have to offer is yours ... and as you rest there for a while ... I wonder if ... only for as long as you want to ... you could allow yourself to examine that pain/discomfort/those sensations you were telling me about ... and allow yourself to *become aware of those sensations as a colour ...* or even a mixture of colours ... and now ... becoming aware of your breathing ... use your out breath to breathe out some of that colour or those colours ... you may find that you prefer to *breathe out just a little of it from around the edges with each out- breath* ... that's right ... or you may prefer to breathe away parts from the core of the sensation ...softening it ... *breathing it away from your body ... breathing it away from your mind ...* you may perhaps *see it flowing away ... the colour floating away as it floats away sensations ... floating away any possible unwanted thoughts at the same time ...drifting ... drifting off ... fading further into the distance ... and ... as you drift ... drifting into a little more ease ...* that's it ... and now *imagine the air around you as having the most wonderful colour of comfort and calm ...* I wonder what it will be ... will it be pale ... translucent perhaps ... or vivid or deep ... or sim-

Begins with an appeal to the kinaesthetic sense

Although, generally speaking, it is a good idea to reframe pain as discomfort, initially it may be crucially important to acknowledge the very really pain that somebody is experiencing. They may very well feel that they are not 'heard' or 'understood' if you do not do this or if you try to reframe too soon.

Use a 'light' tone of voice to encourage floating and drifting

Give lots of pauses

ply have the quality of healing light? Will you catch fleeting glimpses of ethereal colour or will the colour be rich and real as the touch of velvet? And as you breathe in this wonderful calming comfort with each in breath … continuing with each out breath to *breathe out any unwanted colour* … just naturally … breathing, of course, is something that can be done very naturally … breathing *away* discomfort … and breathing *in* the comfort … and I wonder whether you *see the colour of comfort spreading all the way through your body* in any particular direction? Some people notice it beginning at the top of the head and spreading downwards through the body … others notice it beginning at the tips of the toes and spreading upwards to the very top of the head … others still experience it entering the body from all the extremities … the tips of the fingers … the tips of the toes … the scalp … the ears … the nose … others even tell me they *experience the colour as the most amazing sensation of calm* … comforting as it *spreads from the very core of the body like ripples in a pond* … *calming and comforting every single part* … there's no right way … there's no wrong way … whichever way you do *it will be just the perfect way for you* … just getting that sense of easing and soothing all over and all the way through … and while many people find the colour of calm is always constant … others *experience this calm comfort* very slightly differently each time they do this … adapting to every need, every desire … and whichever way you experience it will be so right for you … however you *experience this calm and comforting sensation will be just perfect for you*.

Now reframing pain as discomfort

The use of 'some people' and 'others' offer examples of how they can do it

Merely the mention of the words encourages the awareness of calm in those areas

The phrase '*experience this calm comfort* very slightly differently each time they do this' **seeds the idea of continued practice. Teach self-hypnosis at some point in the trance**

Paint away the pain

Use this script interactively and, when the patient gives you the requested feedback, simply acknowledge it, and continue, using their own words and expressions. These will be far more meaningful and effective than any others imposed upon them.

The underscored examples used here are merely for the purposes of illustration.

People experience all kinds of sensations that somehow don't *seem altogether easy to put into words* ... sometimes, in order that other people can understand the feeling ... sensations can *seem easier to represent in colours and shapes* than to describe in words ... so, how about you discover for yourself how *this can work for you* ... if I were to ask you to *concentrate for a moment on that sensation* and then *tell me what colour it would be*, what would you tell me? Ah, so the colour is <u>red/black</u> ... now if I ask you what shape it is, what will that be? [Pause] I see, it would be a bit like <u>a streak of lightening/triangular shape/bit of a blur</u> ... how interesting ... so what I'd like you to do now is to imagine that there is an easel and canvas/flip chart in front of you and that you have some paints and a paintbrush too and then begin to paint that sensation onto the canvas/paper ... you may even want to mix the paint on a palette to get just the right shade for that <u>streak of lightening/triangular shape/bit of a blur</u> ... tell me, are the edges rough or smooth? ... Oh, the edges are <u>sharp and jagged</u> ... keep painting then ... and, as you do ... tell me more about that <u>red streak of lightning that actually has jagged edges</u> ... is it still or moving? Right, so it's *moving* ... so somehow you've painted in some movement into your picture? Now as you focus on that a bit more, tell me whether it has a temperature, for example is it hot or warm

Embedded command follows the negative

Notice how the tense used here implies the hypothetical 'if I were to ask you to' and 'what would you tell me?' **This makes it easier for someone unused to this type of question to consider such possibilities. Having received an answer, you can continue in the present tense**

or cold … what word would you choose? So, <u>it's like ice</u> … <u>cold as ice</u> … interesting that your paints have special qualities … they can have a wide range of temperatures … … in fact these paints may also have other qualities that you will discover that I have no idea about so can you continue in your own way … in your own time to *paint out that sensation/ those sensations onto the paper … paint them out from you onto the paper* and perhaps find to your surprise … find to your pleasure … that *they are certainly more tolerable there* … some people even say that *although they know the sensation is there, it no longer bothers them in that same old way at all … no longer disturbs them out there …* and while *your body is considering that …* you may *like to think about the colour of comfort and what colour that would be …* Ah, the colour of comfort is <u>pale blue</u> … now here's a very interesting experiment indeed for you to *try out* now … I invite you to paint the <u>streak of lightening a pale blue colour</u> … how do you want to do it? … Do you want to go directly for painting over <u>the red with the pale blue</u> or would you prefer to first 'give it an undercoat of white'? *You do it in the most effective way for you … you could try different ways and find the most comforting and comfortable way for you …* some people have discovered that *it was good to start painting around the edges first …* sort of blurring them out and smoothing everything down and then … as *the sensation of comfort grows* … to move the paintbrush to the centre … whereas other people start right in the centre and *spread the* <u>pale blue</u> *comfort outwards … yes, let me know when that's more comfortable* … interesting, isn't it … now when you're ready let's do some more experimenting … think about which temperature would be most comfortable … do you want to leave it as it was or would you prefer perhaps to <u>warm it up/cool it down</u> a little? … (Now that's interesting …

As therapists we might expect a 'red streak of lightening' **to feel hot. However, sometimes patients will describe the complete opposite and confound all our expectations**

Allow plenty of time between questions for the patient to carry out mental activities and notice the effects

Presupposition 'as *the sensation of comfort grows*'

you're telling me that it already developed a <u>gentle warmth</u> as you painted it <u>pale blue</u> ... and it feels much more comfortable that way? Excellent (shall we leave it like that then?) ... Now just take your time and make any more changes you would like to make to *increase your comfort* ... and isn't it *good to know that you can do this whenever you want to ... you choose all the changes you want to make so that you increase the level of comfort ... remember that there is indeed a harmony between your brain and your body ... and your creative brain can ... and will ... calm and comfort your body in the most amazing of ways.*

Ease away knots of pain and tension

Appeals to the kinaesthetic sense.

And if you were to become aware of any knot-ted feelings anywhere in the mind or body … just imagine taking that knot in your fingers … perhaps you can feel now how it seems to be like a tightly bound ball of wool/string … massage it a little with your fingertips … feel how that warms it a little … softens it slightly … just work it with your fingertips … loosening it … a little more and a little more … till you find the loose end … give it a little tug and notice how it loosens even more when you pull it gently … how it unravels any old, unwanted anxious feelings … how it seems to *relax any unnecessary tension* … a sense of relief as imprisoned/trapped feelings can be set free from that knot and ease their way out and away … away with your breathing … away from the body … away from the mind … away with your breathing … and notice how that seems to *let every muscle go … ease every tiny little muscle fibre … comfort every part of you … soothe every nerve ending in the mind and body* … so much more peaceful now … so much more comfortable now … a sense of relief … a sense of freedom.

Notice how these phrases are giving a sense of taking control. The more control a person feels over pain, generally the easier it is to bear

'a sense of freedom' **picks up on the earlier metaphor of imprisoned feelings being** 'set free' **from the knot**

Pass the parcel

This metaphor has kinaesthetic, visual and general imaginative appeal. It is important to convey to your client that they should continue to use this metaphor at home as a self-hypnosis activity as a means of managing their pain or discomfort whenever they need to do so.

This script includes reference to many different elements of pain, some of which will be more appropriate than others to your particular patient. Take care to read the script ahead of time and omit any that you deem unsuitable for some reason. Your patient may well have some interesting responses to the session and you can, of course, use the metaphor on a subsequent visit making use of different responses arising from your discussion.

Sitting/lying there for a while … becoming even a little more relaxed just listening to my voice … you can allow your mind to *recapture some happy childhood memories* … did you ever have parties? … For birthdays or Christmas or some type of celebration … where you played party games? … I loved those old-fashioned games … really simple ones … like musical chairs … or musical statues or pass the parcel … that was a nice one … you know the one where there was a small present wrapped up in sheet after sheet of wrapping paper … and you had to sit in a circle on the floor and pass round the parcel from one to another while the music played … and when the music stopped and *you* had the parcel … you had to tear the paper off and then continue passing it around … with different layers being removed until eventually the parcel was so small there was only one layer of paper left … it was such a good feeling when it was your turn and you could unwrap that last layer and you could claim your present … do you remember that feeling? … Sometimes there were other little presents along the way that would drop out into your lap as you tore the paper off as you removed another layer … quite unexpectedly … such a lovely surprise.

Insert some other celebration if more culturally appropriate

Seeds the idea of the 'pass the parcel' game and, hopefully, revivifies pleasant memories

Have you ever found that … as you *let your mind drift back to old pleasant memories* you surprise yourself how easy it is to let the years drift away and you can *be amazed how completely you are right back in the memory* … right back in the moment and you can *enjoy the moment all over again … you can really have some very good experiences this way* … so I invite you to join me in a game of pass the parcel now … I have an idea for a slight variation. … Have a look at the parcel … I'm not sure whether it's wrapped in brown paper or brightly coloured wrapping paper or even newspaper … or maybe … as you take off the layers one by one … you will discover a mixture of all of these. This variation of the game is one where the parcel is made up of the pain/discomfort that you told me about and … as you probably know … pain/discomfort is made up of many layers …so it seems really quite appropriate to *peel away those layers* … don't you think? … Everybody experiences things a little differently but you might find that there are layers of tension and anxiety there just aching to be released … so I think it's your turn now … to take the parcel in your hands and unwrap that layer … yes … and at the same time … use your breathing and breathe out … let the tension go … now I don't know if you want to unwrap the parcel very carefully and deliberately or whether you prefer to tear/rip off that layer of paper … I only know that as you do it, it will make a significant difference to the way you are able to relax away unwanted tense feelings … relax away anxious thoughts … feel yourself relaxing more deeply now … that's right … I think you have *time to tear off another piece now* … and you may notice that there is a very special box beside you where you can put all the paper you've removed … relaxing deeper and deeper … feeling already perhaps a sense of relief as you pass the parcel on now … a sense of relief continuing with your breathing as you await your next turn … that's it … relaxing even deeper now with the sound of my voice.

Revivifies pleasant childhood memories

Invites more vivid imagination of the parcel

Begins to educate the client about elements and perceptions of pain. Mention those which have particular relevance to the person in front of you

Offers a double bind choice … whichever way they unwrap the parcel, carefully or otherwise, a layer is being removed

And continuing to relax as you patiently await your turn ... intrigued to discover which layers you can *peel away next* ... perhaps you can become aware of any possible memory that you might have stored of painful/unpleasant/aching/dull/burning sensations that you've experienced in the past ... realising now ... possibly for the first time ... that dwelling on the memory of that previous experience can actually ... for some people ... be responsible for increasing their level of pain or discomfort in the moment ... so as the parcel is handed back to you now ... I'm wondering if you will *surprise yourself as you* unwrap *the next sheet of paper* ... and you find that you are *peeling away* feelings from the past ... perhaps some feelings that you had no conscious idea were there ... perhaps others that you had been aware you were holding onto for some reason ... but now feeling *free to release them with your breathing* ... *even ... doing it all at the unconscious level* ...and *experience a sense of relief as you let them disperse now* ... and of course ... when we talk of the past ... it can refer to years gone by ... or merely days or hours or even just minutes ago ... just peeling away the layers now ...and letting go anything from the past that could be harmful in any way. ... How does it feel in your hands, I wonder, as you choose to tear away that layer? ... How does it feel in your mind? Is there a surprise gift of a sudden realisation that ... actually ... you can choose *NOT* to 'squirrel away' negative past 'feeling-memories' ... you can *consign them to the past* and delight in a freer, more comfortable present? ... How does that feel in the body? ... Maybe it will surprise you that *letting go of an out-of-date thought can change so much?* ... And allowing your breathing to help *relax yourself deeper and deeper still* ... and feeling my voice take you deeper and deeper relaxed and calm ... relaxed and calm and more comfortable now. So ... time to pass the parcel on now and *enjoy the rest* even a little more ... maybe watching others peel away layers ... curious to see what they find.

Remembered Pain
Presupposition that layers exist

Use the client's own expressions here

The use of 'for *some* people' **can help to bypass resistance**

'*even doing it all at the unconscious level*' **allows a sense of release even if the patient doesn't know consciously what is being released**

Covers all aspects of the past; recent or time from long ago

'feeling my voice' **a deliberate mixing of the senses**

I wonder if they're finding the 'layer of anticipation'? ... This is a different layer that consists of what people *expect* to feel ... possibly because of their own past experience ... or because of careless words from other people ... sometimes words from professionals can be misleading or sometimes open to misinterpretation by a patient ... and it's very common to let other people influence us quite unfairly ... these are the people who are quick to exaggerate their own experience (think how sometimes a woman who has been through a difficult birth can seem almost to delight in terrifying other pregnant women with her tale of woe ... and *finally what a relief it can be* for this new mother to discover that her own experience of childbirth is something so wondrous and joyful that she can *bear those sensations with equanimity with the focus of her mind on something ... or indeed someone ... else entirely*) ... Time to take the parcel back now and ... yes, it's your turn again to *remove another layer* ... so notice what happens as you begin tearing off this bit of paper ... does it *release any negative/ unhelpful expectations* so they seem to drift up and away almost as though you could *see as well as feel them lifting off you* ...deciding to choose your own thoughts and expectations so that they *increase your comfort* ... understanding that you really can *choose your thoughts to improve your mood and increase your comfort*.

Anticipated Pain

Embedded commands

Use your voice to emphasise the word 'choose'

There can be emotional layers too that may *be best discarded ... or at least temporarily stored elsewhere* ... did you already know ... (or is this new to you?) ... that if a person is sad or unhappy that their perception of pain/a negative sensation will be far stronger? Now, of course I know that there are occasions and events that we face in our lives that can be deeply sad ... tragic even ... and I wouldn't try to pretend that this is not so ... and ... at the same time as acknowledging this ... I wonder if ... moment by moment ... you could allow some of those feelings

Emotional Pain

It's useful to point out that you are not trying to pretend that sadness doesn't exist

to *rest for a while ... rest aside for a while* as you *take the time you need to find the resources inside* and *recoup the energy* to *cope with/manage this experience (as you recover) now.* So ... as it's your turn once again ... can you be very gentle this time as you remove some more wrapping ... glancing down beside you again at that very special box/container ... it can occur to you that this would be a good place to store any unhelpful emotion/sadness/unhappiness that you've uncovered where it can rest safely ... as you *rest too ... comfortably now ... to regain the strength you need* ... knowing that ... if you need to and if you want to ... you can return to this emotion at a time when *you are stronger and can deal with things more resourcefully* ... for the moment the feelings can rest safely in the box/container and *you can rest calmly* ... knowing they are there ... but safely *on the outside* of you ... and finding a little comfort ... and a little more comfort ... and a little more comfort still.

Omit *'as you recover'* **if inappropriate**

This gives them somewhere to store their emotional pain 'outside of them' where it doesn't compound their physical pain. It may be important for them to grieve over a loss for example, but a 'storage place' gives them the opportunity to do this at a time when they are feeling stronger and more able to do so. Be aware that they may be mourning the loss of their physical strength and health and this loss should not be underestimated

And of course you may know ... or suspect ... that there are other layers too that you want to unwrap and choose to let free ... layers that I have no idea about at the moment ... (nor do I need to know) ... so I am going to remain quiet for a while now while you continue unwrapping and letting go ... increasing your comfort ... until you let me know that you have unwrapped everything and found the special little box in the centre waiting there for you. Let me know when you've found it but don't unwrap it yet.

Other Unknown Personal Elements Of Pain

Stay quiet until they signal they have finished

So here is your gift ... you have many choices now ... you may choose to open it now if you want to ... or you may choose to take it with you and open it another time ... or you may choose simply to carry it with you and allow your unconscious mind to find exactly the right time to surprise you in the nicest of ways by opening it for you ... or it may be that one day you simply realise your present was the gift of a comfortable absence of something you no longer

Optional Ending 1

Intentional confusion

needed or wanted ... or it could be a gradual aware-ness of unawareness of something that has faded into the background as of absolutely no importance to you at all ... whatever ... wherever ... whenever or however it happens can be a special gift for you.

So here is your gift ... it is a precious gift from your unconscious mind ... that may remain a mystery to your conscious mind as to how it works ... but over the next few hours/days/weeks and months (as appropriate) you have a sense of being comforted ... physically ... emotionally and mentally ... you will become aware that you are feeling stronger ... you are feeling more optimistic ... you have an inner sense of equanimity/calm/being able to cope with anything and anybody.

Optional Ending 2

Include the patient's desired states and resources

The words 'any' **and** 'body' **are intentionally separated out here**

Go to a suitable trance reorientation

161

Layers of pain

This script is adapted from *Pass the parcel* using the same metaphor of *Layers of pain*, with kinaesthetic, visual and general imaginative appeal, but it doesn't include the idea of the children's party game, which for some people will be less appropriate. It is important to convey to your client that they should continue to use this metaphor at home as a self-hypnosis activity as a means of managing their pain or discomfort whenever they need to do so.

This script includes reference to many different elements of pain, some of which will be more relevant than others to your particular patient. Take care to read the script ahead of time and omit any elements that you deem unsuitable for any reason. Your patient may well have some interesting responses to the session and you can, of course, use the metaphor on a subsequent visit, making use of different responses arising from your discussion.

Sitting/lying there for a while … becoming even a little more relaxed just listening to my voice … I wonder if *you are prepared to allow your mind to focus on that pain* that you told me about … actually to do the opposite of what you had been trying to do before … *distract yourself from the pain*, that is … and it might be that … as you take a little while to *explore just what is going on there* … you'll be surprised to *discover something meaningful* … and indeed quite useful … to you.

> This may surprise the patient as they are being encouraged to (temporarily) focus on the pain instead of being asked to ignore it. Surprise is often a useful tactic in trance and just 'being given permission' to focus on the pain can actually be a relief, particularly if their previous attempts to distract themselves have seemed impossibly difficult

Have you ever found before that … as you *learned something new* … it gave you a means of dealing with something that was surprisingly effective? So as you focus on that pain/discomfort that you told me about … let's think about just what it consists of … I don't know if you already know that pain/discomfort is made up of many layers … some that we know about consciously and some that we only recognize at the unconscious level … one layer of course is the physical sensation itself, but there are several others

> This question hopefully revivifies a previously useful reference experience but, even if it doesn't succeed in doing this, it will seed the idea that a 'surprisingly effective way' of dealing with pain may exist

... sometimes many others ... so it seems really quite appropriate to examine them more closely ... see what else is nestling in there that possibly doesn't need to be there ... and perhaps even *peel away some of those layers* ... don't you think? ... Now, everybody experiences things a little differently ... some people *see the layers* ... like layers of an onion that you can *peel away* ... some people think of layers of clothing worn on a cold winter's day which ... once inside the house ... you begin to take off as *you no longer need them* ... some people feel the layers while others just *get a sense of the layers being present in some way* ... but you might well find that there are layers of tension and anxiety just aching to be released ... so in whichever way is right for you ... you can begin gently to lift up the first layer and find the tension ... yes, that's right ... and at the same time ... use your breathing and breathe out ... let the tension go ... now I don't know if you want to continue by lifting the layer very carefully and deliberately or whether you prefer to tear/rip it off ... I only know that as you do it, it will make a significant difference to the way you are able to *relax away unwanted tense feelings* ... *relax away anxious thoughts* ... *feel yourself relaxing more deeply now* ... that's right ... and when you're ready ... you can remove another layer still ... and you may notice that there is a very special box/container beside you where you can put anything you want to ... just relaxing deeper and deeper ... feeling already perhaps a sense of relief as you *enjoy the rest* ... a sense of relief continuing with your breathing as you take all the time you need to *relax more comfortably now* ... that's it ... relaxing even deeper now with the sound of my voice.

And continuing to relax as you begin to wonder about other layers ... intrigued to discover which layers you will find and *can peel away next* ... perhaps you can become aware of any possible memory that you might have stored of painful/unpleasant/aching/dull/burning sensations that you've experienced in

Truism

'some people see or think' **suggests different perceptions they may find useful**

Offers a double bind choice ... whichever way they lift the layer, carefully or otherwise, it is being removed

Note the ambiguity of *'enjoy the rest'* (**rest meaning relaxation**) **or** (**rest meaning the remainder of the session**)

Remembered Pain

'*which* layers' **presupposes layers exist**

Use the client's own expressions here

the past ... realising now ... possibly for the first time ... that dwelling on the memory of that previous experience can actually ... for some people ... be responsible for increasing their level of pain or discomfort in the moment ... so as you *move onto the next layer now* ... I'm wondering if you will *surprise yourself as you* remove it ... and perhaps find that you are *peeling away* feelings from the past ... possibly even feelings that you had no conscious idea were there ... and perhaps others that you had been aware you were holding onto for some reason ... but now, feeling *free to release them ... even doing it all at the unconscious level ... with your breathing* ... and *experience a wonderful sense of relief as you let them disperse now* ... and of course ... when we talk of the past ... it can refer to years gone by ... or merely days or hours or even just minutes ago ... just peeling away the layers now ...and letting go anything from the past that could be harmful in any way ... How does it feel in your hands, I wonder, as you *choose to remove that layer*? ... How does it feel in your mind? Is there a surprising sudden realisation that ... actually ... you can choose *NOT* to 'squirrel away' negative past 'feeling-memories' ... you can *consign them to the past* and delight in a freer, more comfortable present? ... How does that feel in the body? ... Maybe it will surprise you that *letting go of an out-of-date thought can change so much?* ... And allowing your breathing to help *relax yourself deeper and deeper still* ... and feeling my voice take you deeper and deeper relaxed and calm ... *relaxed and calm and more comfortable now*. So ... time to take a small break now and *enjoy the rest even a little more* ... maybe allowing your imagination to *become really curious* to see what it will find next.

Will it be the 'layer of anticipation' perhaps? ... This is a different layer that consists of what people *expect* to feel ... possibly because of their own past experience ... or because of careless words from other people ... sometimes words from professionals can

The use of 'for *some* people' **can help to bypass resistance**

'even doing it all at the unconscious level' **allows the sense of release even if the patient doesn't know consciously what is being released**

Anticipated Pain

be misleading or sometimes open to misinterpretation by a patient ... and it's very common to let other people influence us quite unfairly ... these are the ones who are quick to exaggerate their own experience (think how sometimes a woman who has been through a difficult birth can seem almost to delight in terrifying other pregnant women with her tale of woe ... and *finally what a relief it can be* for this new mother to discover that her own experience of childbirth is something so wondrous and joyful that she can *bear those sensations with equanimity with the focus of her mind on something ... or indeed someone ... else entirely).*

This metaphor may have less relevance to a male patient. If so, omit it or choose a more neutral example

Do you think it's time to *remove another layer*? ... so notice what happens as you begin ... does it *release any negative/unhelpful expectations* so they seem to drift up and away almost as though you could *see as well as feel them lifting off you* ...deciding to choose your own thoughts and expectations so that they *increase your comfort* ... understanding that *you really can choose your thoughts to improve your mood and increase your comfort ... choose to empower yourself as you relax even deeper now* ... deeper than you thought you could ... and you could (couldn't you?)... *do that right now.*

Note the ambiguity of *'do that right now'.* It could refer to relaxing more deeply or empowering yourself or, of course, both!

Emotional Pain

There can be emotional layers too that may *be best discarded ... or at least temporarily stored elsewhere* ... did you already know ... (or is this new to you?) ... that if a person is sad or unhappy that their perception of pain/a negative sensation will be far stronger? Now, of course I know that there are occasions and events that we face in our lives that can be deeply sad ... tragic even ... and I wouldn't try to pretend that this is not so ... and ... at the same time as acknowledging this ... I wonder if ... moment by moment ... you could allow some of those feelings to *rest for a while ... rest aside for a while* as you

It's useful to point out that you are not trying to pretend that sadness doesn't exist

take the time you need to find the resources inside and *recoup the energy* to *cope with/manage this experience (as you recover) now.* So … being very gentle as you uncover more layers and glancing down beside you again at that very special box/ container … it can occur to you that this would be a good place to put any unhelpful emotion/sadness/ unhappiness that you've uncovered where it can rest safely … as you *rest too … comfortably now … to regain the strength you need* … knowing that … if you need to and if you want to … you can return to this emotion at a time when *you are stronger and can deal with things more resourcefully* … for the moment the feelings can rest safely in the box/container and you can rest calmly … knowing they are there … but safely on the outside of you and finding a little comfort … and a little more comfort … and a little more comfort still.

Omit *'as you recover'* **if inappropriate**

This gives them somewhere to store their emotional pain 'outside of them' where it doesn't compound their physical pain. It may be important for them to grieve over a loss for example, but a 'storage place' gives them the opportunity to do this at a time when they are feeling stronger and more able to do so. Be aware that they may be mourning the loss of their physical strength and health and this loss shouldn't be underestimated

And of course you may know … or suspect … that there are other layers too that you want to uncover and choose to let free … so I am going to remain quiet for a while now while you continue uncovering … removing and letting go … increasing your comfort … until you let me know that you have completed everything you want to do today. [Pause] Thank you … Good job/well done.

Other Unknown Personal Elements of Pain

Stay quiet until they signal they have finished

So today you have begun a process of letting go of unhelpful, unwanted thoughts, feelings and sensations and this will continue at many levels … and … the great thing is … that once you have *let go of those unwanted thoughts and emotions* … you receive/gain something very positive in their place … you receive a gift which will improve your experience of life … sometimes in a quite unexpected way … you may find that your unconscious mind finds *special occasions* to surprise you in the nicest of ways … or it may *be a growing awareness* over a period of time of a sense of being comforted … physically … emotionally and mentally … you will become aware that you are feeling stronger … you are feeling more

Presupposition you will 'let go'

optimistic … you have an inner sense of equanimity/ calm … becoming more able to *cope with anything and anybody* or it may be that one day you simply realise your gift is simply a comfortable absence of something you no longer needed or wanted … or it could be a gradual awareness of unawareness of something that has faded into the background as of absolutely no importance to you at all … whatever … wherever … whenever or however it happens can be a special gift for you.

Go to a suitable trance reorientation

The words 'any' **and** 'body' **are intentionally separated out here to emphasize the patient's ability to cope with any discomfort experienced in the body**

Leave the pain beside you

Prepare for a medical procedure, for example changes of burns dressings, invasive procedures such as biopsies, scopes or dental surgery.

This script, which deals with a state of *temporary dissociation from pain*, has been adapted from *Leave the pain beside the court* in the *Sport and Performance* section.

Now you are feeling more comfortably relaxed ... so comfortable and relaxed that there are times when you're hardly aware of your body at all ... totally absorbed in drifting into an even more creative and receptive state of mind ... you can begin to address the purpose of your visit ... to find a way for you to *have this procedure carried out with a good sense of calm and comfort throughout (and with the very least discomfort/sensation possible)* ... your body's natural endorphins flowing through your body and keeping it very comfortable indeed ... and isn't it reassuring to know that in the state of hypnosis your mind and body can work amazingly well in harmony to *allow this to occur* ... just as you want it to ... just as you need it to ... I expect that you know ... (or is this the first time that you've heard of it?) ... that patients have used the state of hypnosis to have operations/dental treatment quite painlessly with no anaesthetic at all ... and I'm sure you already know ... even without the help of hypnosis ... how people can use the mind to *direct attention away from the body* ... you may well have done this consciously or unconsciously yourself in a very ordinary way ... somehow, for example ... able to *convince your body that it had enough energy* and it had enough power to *continue an activity even though you were really tired because what you were doing really needed to be done* ... and then again, think about those people who *carry out quite amazing things on occasion* ... we've all read about cases where a person

Restates the goal, which concentrates the mind, but also provides the opportunity to embed appropriate commands. Some people may find it easier to accept the bracketed suggestion

Illustrates the power of hypnosis

An everyday example of how we can use our minds to influence our bodies in a positive way

is able to *find a kind of superhuman strength* to lift a vehicle and release someone trapped beneath it … or someone badly injured has managed to carry a companion to safety … temporarily completely unaware of their own feelings … and because of the power of the mind … were able to *do this safely* so this is an ability *we all have inside us when we really need it* … and you have told me that you really need to have this procedure for your overall health and well-being … that's it's important for you to have it and that you *really want to go in and do it calmly and comfortably and stay completely in control.*

Earlier you told me that you were frightened of pain … so let's have a think about pain … in a certain way of course it's there for a very good reason … one of the very useful purposes of an unpleasant sensation is to alert us to the fact that part of our body could be in danger … but actually in your case *you know* very well that the upcoming procedure is happening for a very good reason and you have already made an informed decision that *you want to accept the treatment* because it is going to help you get better/ improve your health/prevent your becoming (more) ill … and … as you have been told that it is important/ crucial for you to have this treatment … *it is, in fact, very safe* for you to *ignore the discomfort/sensation* … *it's even safe* for you not to be aware of it at all and *you can do this* in a rather unusual way … I'd like you to become aware of the part of you that knows how to experience pain … let yourself imagine it as a personality in its own right … maybe *you can see it* or just *become aware of it in some way* … and you could have a bit of a chat with it … just silently in your mind now … and you can of course use your own words to *do it* … just explain that you fully respect its primary purpose … nevertheless … as you have definitely decided to *have this treatment for your own well-being* … ask it to *take a break while you are having the treatment* … allow you to *feel calm and comfortable all the way through* while it does a very important but slightly different job for

Reminds them of amazing feats that human beings can achieve through the power of the mind and also embeds commands

Adapt this to the circumstances of your client

Acknowledge their fear of pain. It's certainly at the forefront of their mind or they wouldn't be with you. First explain a positive purpose of pain as a warning of danger. Then reframe by pointing out that, as they are not in danger, they can safely ignore it

Dissociation and informal parts work

you ... OK, just do that now ... mentally and silently and let me know when you've done it. [Pause] OK, good. So the very moment the procedure begins, *that part that feels sensation can float out of your body* and sit there beside the chair/bed/beside you ... just watching you to check you are OK ... its role is to *experience any possible discomfort **outside** your body* so that *nothing bothers you at all ... nothing disturbs you in any way* ... that part sitting over there can experience any necessary sensations ... so that *you* don't have to ... it can *do it right over there ... completely away from you* ... and allow you to *receive your treatment comfortably* ... you will know it's happening ... and ... *you can remain entirely comfortable throughout* ... and that part sitting over there has two responsibilities ... one is to experience any sensations outside of your body so that *you yourself don't have to be aware of it at all* ... and the second responsibility is to be aware that ... at any time when you might truly need to be alerted to any possible danger to yourself ... its job would be to step back into your body and give you a warning so you could safeguard yourself ... other than that, its job is to protect you from discomfort ... so just take another moment or two just silently within yourself ... to check that 'your pain part' is agreeable to this plan and then we will move to the final part of the session. [Pause]

Excellent. All that remains to do here with me now ... and also for you to do every day when you're at home ... *and then again in the hospital/dental surgery/treatment room* ... is for you to *imagine that you are watching a film of you* ... can you see it? Good ... look at you so calm and confident there and ... as you do ... notice how *there is a part of you that is floating up and out of you ... floating right over there to sit down and make itself very comfortable indeed on the chair/bed/the cupboard* ... (what does that part look like, I wonder?) as it settles down to watch you *behave absolutely magnificently* while it does whatever it needs to do to *keep*

'the part that feels sensation can float out of your body' **encourages dissociation**

'that part sitting over there' **encourages further dissociation**

More dissociation

Gives the part a 'safety net'

Reframes pain as discomfort

Repetition of the positive imagery at home is essential for reinforcement

Observation of the dissociation

'what does that part look like?' **encourages further dissociation** *you safe … your body's natural endorphins flowing through your body keep you comfortable and strong … keep you calm and at ease all the way through … look at you … nothing bothers you … nothing disturbs you … you are completely at ease … you are magnificent!*

And once its job is done … so amazingly well … that part of you that has been on guard … experiencing any necessary temporary sensations for you on the outside … so as to keep you as comfortable as can be … will automatically float back into your body … so that all parts of you are fully integrated … your mind and body in harmony … now feeling positive and pleased with a very successful outcome … and also comfortably reassured that you have a part of you … that can keep you safe, both by letting appropriate sensations indicate that something needs attention if and when necessary and also … at your own request … by protecting you from unwanted sensation when it is safe for it to do so … a very special ability indeed.

So now it's time for you to *reorient to the room* … every part of you understanding its very own special role for you … keeping you just as comfortable as can be … isn't it good to *know that your unconscious mind and your body can do this together … knowing exactly when and which parts to let rest or even sleep for a while …* allowing your body's own innate forces to produce their natural calming and comforting endorphins while doing their wonderful healing work … gently returning to conscious awareness of *how much more rested you feel … how much more comfortable you feel … how much you have calmed and taken control of your thoughts* … gently comfortably coming back now … with *that sense of optimism … in a rather unusual way … being experienced in your body as well as in your mind …* a strong sense of being *focused on positive ideas and experiences … a feeling of being uplifted and supported* wherever you are … whenever you're

Reintegration of parts

Reminder that 'this part' can carry out two functions. It can use painful sensations as an indication that something needs attention but it can also allow dissociation from pain if and when it is safe to do so

This ending, to be used after any *pain relief script*, can also be found in the Trance Reorientations section

Some parts can be rested or allowed to sleep, e.g. the parts which experience chronic pain or parts which have been temporarily dissociated

Presuppositions of greater well-being and optimism

there ... whomever you're with or simply when you're comfortably and easily enjoying your own company ... that's it ... refreshed and well rested ... welcome back.

Float off to somewhere pleasant

Dissociate the mind away from the body.

Use any induction and deepener with suggestions for feelings of lightness rather than heaviness.

And in this very/more comfortable and relaxed state of altered awareness ... where your mind has become remarkably creative and unbound by conscious parameters ... I'm going to invite you to let your mind *float off* to somewhere where you can *enjoy the most pleasing of daydreams/memories/ fantasies* ... it can be any delightful experience you like ... you may find that you *drift off temporarily away from the body to some special place* where you've been before ... somewhere that has wonder- ful memories that make you smile ... images that delight your senses ... feelings of such comfort and ease ... thoughts that *entrance you* ... somewhere that gladdens the heart as you experience this.

Or could it be that you *float off* to some fantasy land where you can *enjoy exploring somewhere new* ... discovering charming places where you will *create wonderful memories* that you can safely *return to again and again in your mind* whenever you want to *experience something quite splendid/exquisite/ lovely* ... is this some place where you are happy in your own company or are there people with you that you have specially chosen to have accompany you? Wherever you are ... comfortably familiar or intrigu- ingly new ... your mind is so completely absorbed in this place of intense fascination/comfort and ease/ haven of peace ... that it can temporarily be hardly aware of your body at all ... you can allow your body to rest for a while ... soothed by comforting endor- phins ... as your mind enjoys its travels/daydream/ the experience.

You may use a prearranged experience or simply leave the unconscious mind to come up with the most appropriate one at the time. Even if mentioning somewhere prearranged, it is useful to allow the unconscious the prerogative to change its mind!

And you can be here for as long as you like ... enjoying your unconscious mind's ability to expand or contract time as suits you best ... at times a long time can seem like a very short time and a short time can seem like a long time ... the important thing is that this is your choice to enjoy time in the way that is perfect for you.

Brief suggestions for time distortion. You can find a longer script in the *Miscellaneous* section

Go to more therapeutic suggestions or to a suitable trance reorientation as appropriate

Variations, Adaptations and Recommendations

This dissociation script could be used as a short-term means of 'mentally floating out of the body' for a medical or dental procedure or it could be used as a way to give temporary relief from chronic pain. In the first case, be certain to integrate all parts during the trance reorientation.

In the second case, you might like to include suggestions for the part to bring back only comfortable feelings as it reintegrates and also to emphasize its ability to float out safely whenever it needs to experience some relief from physical sensation. Clearly it would be useful to teach this as part of a self-hypnosis procedure so the patient could use it at will.

When using the metaphor with a patient who suffers from intense chronic pain it will be more appropriate to choose the option of 'more comfortable' in the opening line, 'And in this very comfortable/more comfortable and relaxed state of altered awareness'. If not, the patient may feel their pain has not been sufficiently acknowledged and this can cause an unwillingness to participate fully in the experience.

Antenatal, Childbirth, Post-natal

Take care of your health: considerations

Some women may request help in keeping to a healthy diet, stopping smoking, taking regular appropriate light exercise (including pelvic floor exercise), keeping alcohol within limits or simply taking enough rest. All of the above would be appropriate areas in which you can help pregnant women through positive suggestion but remember that, unless you are qualified to deal with pregnancy care, you should avoid giving advice. Rather, you should encourage them to check out their concerns with their health care professional.

Morning sickness refers to the nausea and vomiting that some women have when they become pregnant. It may be caused by the sudden increase in hormones or perhaps lower blood sugar during early pregnancy. It tends to go away after the first few weeks but each individual is different so there are no set times for everybody. Emotional stress, fatigue, travelling, or certain foods can make the problem worse and although nausea is more common in the morning, it can occur at any time of the day or night.

It is always important to check that your client has been assured that the morning sickness being experienced may be safely ignored before treating with hypnotherapy.

Cope with morning sickness

Relaxing even more deeply now and being pleasantly aware of an increasing sense of comfort and
ease ... you may find yourself also becoming aware
of a growing sense of pleasant absorption in your
own inner world ... mentally and physically at ease
with yourself ... and in some unusual kind of a way
... finding times when you *feel so comfortable in
yourself at an inner level* ... that *you can be almost
completely unaware of yourself at an outer level*
... (and that does seem unusual, does it not?) ...
but that is one of the amazing effects of hypnotic
relaxation ... hypnotic thinking ... hypnotic feeling
... you can *experience things very differently* all at
the same time ... you can know of course that your
body is there but at the same time *you can choose
to be in your inner world and be scarcely aware of
your physical self at all.*

**Suggests that the hypnotic
state allows a different
experience of self**

Just as ... in the same way ... the 'thinking part' of
you can know that something called morning sickness could exist ... while your physical part *can have
almost no awareness of it at all. In a physical and
emotional sense it seems almost irrelevant to you*
because you always take care of your health and eat
healthily and well ... at first you tend to eat smaller
meals more frequently and you can *feel very satisfied
with that* ... and when you need to do so ... you will
adjust your diet according to the needs of your body
and the advice of your practitioner/midwife/health
care professional ... but actually your body is wise
... it usually knows what it needs and what is good
... what is good for you and what is good for your
baby ... you *listen to professional advice and you
listen to the wisdom of your body ... the important
thing is that you stay positive and you stay calm and
you fully enjoy your pregnancy.*

**Hypnotic thinking allows
conscious knowledge of
nausea with little, if any,
physical awareness of it**

I am sure you're aware that *your mind and body
together have extraordinary abilities both in your
waking and your sleeping state* ... and working

in harmony in the *hypnotic* state … these abilities are so enhanced that they can produce the most amazing effects … a calm and happy thought in the mind for example can create powerful endorphins in the body … that *calm and settle the tummy* … sometimes spreading gradually down through the body and sometimes swiftly filling *the area with what seems like an inner soothing balm … providing immediate, welcome relief … some people think of cooling streams or lakes … and others think of a setting sun … why don't you experiment in your imagination now and discover which is the most calming, comforting and effective image for you?*

Emphasize the word *'hypnotic'*

And … as you become so absorbed in your inner world at times … you will find that the outer world seems to fly past … and in this hypnotic state … you can *strengthen that unconscious ability to become so absorbed in your inner world* … as and when you want to … whenever, of course, that it's safe for you to do so … that you *take yourself off in your mind to somewhere special and intensely absorbing* … and you *feel very content to be there and let time fly past taking any hint of unsettled sensations with it* … one young woman told me of how … when she wanted to mentally absent herself from her body … she would always take herself off to a beautiful beach/garden/mountain/stream somewhere in her mind … and sit quietly and ponder which name she would choose for her baby … would it be Evie or Ella or perhaps Olivia for a girl … or Jack or Tom or Matthew or Ben for a boy? … She said she got endless delight whenever she thought about it … visualising her baby growing up with this name or that name … wondering if it would suit them … wondering whether they would like the name they'd been given.

A common source of fascination with expectant mothers

So you too … from now on will discover to your delight … that you can *speed up any possible unsettled time … so it will seem insignificant* … as you drift off/transport yourself to your special place … where *you are totally absorbed and comfortable* … and … whenever *you feel really well and your stomach is calm and settled* … this time *will slow down* and you can really *enjoy those calm and settled feelings* for so much longer … and *you tend to be very aware all the time of the time when you're feeling fine* … you *notice how well you feel and you notice how well you look* … (and *there must be something very special about you*)… since your friends … and even people you don't know so well … seem to *notice and comment on how well you look.*

So why not take a little time now … which might seem like a long time … *to see in your mind's eye how things are going to be* … *getting better every day* … *see yourself looking so good* … feeling so fit … going about your daily routine … look at the smile on your face … waking up feeling well rested after a good night's sleep … *you really do sleep so well* … feeling good … looking forward to your day … see yourself just naturally reaching out for a cracker/ plain biscuit … *calm and settled inside* … getting up gently … knowing *it's going to be a very good day indeed* … you remember without even consciously thinking about it to *eat little and often* as your mind has learned its lesson very well … *it speeds up any possible time when you could be feeling a bit down so you can cope with it easily and calmly* … *you can bear any possible unsettled sensations because you know they will pass very quickly* … *that's right* … *and your mind will slow down the positive time so you can enjoy every minute* … delighting in the knowledge that you are going to have a baby … how wonderful … and when you look back … you will know that you *put in place everything necessary to care for your health* … *feel comfortable and settled* … *take everything in your stride and enjoy this very special time as you nurture your baby until he or she is ready to be born.*

Personalise this. Have them visualise eating appealing food with a completely settled stomach

Go to a suitable trance reorientation or add in further appropriate suggestions

Variations, Adaptations and Recommendations

Quick reminder suggestions for coping with morning sickness for inclusion in other scripts if desired:

- Stay positive/Stay calm/Keep an outward focus.
- You can bear it as it will pass.
- You can be aware of it mentally but physically it won't bother you at all.
- Becoming less and less aware of it with each passing day.
- Time distortion: time passes more quickly during periods of nausea.
- Having suffered morning sickness previously has no bearing on this particular pregnancy.
- Visualisation of eating appropriately and feeling well.

Bonding with your unborn baby

This script may be used alone or in conjunction with other antenatal short scripts as appropriate. The script includes a gentle relaxation induction followed by the breathing in of 'pure light' and a visualisation of the perfectly formed baby. This in itself is sufficient to induce a light trance state but, if desired, it can be prefaced by any other gentle induction technique. After the visualisation of bonding with the baby, there is a teaching process of light self-hypnosis to be used at home. This also serves to deepen the trance state of your client and so increases their receptivity to the ego strengthening which follows.

How nice it is to take some time for yourself to relax ... take the weight off your feet and let your eyelids gently close ... make yourself very comfortable and check that you *feel well supported as you relax* ... both here at this time ... and later too at home when you *choose to return to this experience again and again until the moment when you hold your baby in your arms* ... sitting here now being aware first of the comfort and support (of the cushions) at your back ... then, your sides ... your legs ... your feet ... now check the feelings of comfort as you *relax your head and your neck into the cushions behind you* ... be aware of that sense of relief as your head sinks into those cushions/that pillow ... relaxing the muscles in your head and your neck ... that's it ... now relaxing the muscles in your shoulders ... and notice ... as you do so ... how your shoulders seem to *sink gently down* into your arms ... now letting the arms relax so that *any possible tension drifts down through your elbows* ... down through your wrists ... down through your hands and out through your fingertips ... finding just enough energy to let your hands gently rest on your stomach/abdomen ... just finding the most comfortable position for you and ... of course ... do know, that if you want to shift your position at any time to *increase your comfort* ... you will *do this naturally and easily* ... and I don't know whether you will *experience this as a single wave of comfort* that flows all over your body or whether

In late pregnancy it is best for mothers to avoid lying flat on their back as this can increase the risk of fainting. Ideally position your client so she is either sitting with her legs and feet supported, or lying comfortably on her side

Embedded commands

A presupposition which offers them a choice of two suggestions which are equally desirable

180

it will *seem more like little ripples of comfort easing their way all down and all the way through your body* … but you can *allow it to happen in just the right way for you* … in just the right way for your baby … interesting (isn't it?) … how sometimes when you *relax your body so completely,* your baby senses this and relaxes along with you … both of you enjoying this peaceful time together … and how … at other times … your baby simply appreciates the peace and calm of your body and delights in the freedom to move around easily … already discovering the wonder of his or her own beautifully developing body … as of course you too can wonder at the little miracle/this precious little being inside you that is developing and growing stronger and stronger every day.

And you can *take some time out now to enjoy a very special time together* … imagine, if you will, that the air around you is filled with a pure, shining light and … as you breathe it in … the light seems to shine all through you … so that you seem to be glowing with light and love *… it increases your inner tranquillity* … and each in breath also seems to enhance all of your senses … you *become sensitive in the best of ways* … sensitive to inner sounds and sights and sensations … beginning to *get a sense of this amazing bond with your baby* … seeing in your mind's eye this tiny little being … this beautiful baby that is yours … floating inside you … imagining gently caressing them … sensing your baby's delight at your delicate touch … or perhaps simply caressing them with your eyes … seeing and feeling every tiny little perfectly formed part … how amazing! … And can you *let yourself become aware* that … through your enhanced sensitivity today … you are creating this wonderful way to *communicate with your baby* … you can use your breathing to breathe the feelings of love …each breath conveying that love …and you can use words and the words will be received through their senses … you can tell them how much you want them … you can tell them how much you are looking forward to meeting them … you can

A deepener with suggestions to heighten sensitivity in order to bond with the baby in the womb

Auditory

Visual

Kinaesthetic

Presupposition of enhanced sensitivity

Not every woman has a fully developed instinct on mother–baby bonding. These suggestions can help a prospective mother develop a sense of how to communicate with her unborn child

reassure them that until that time comes ... you will give them all the nourishment they need so they continue to grow and develop into a healthy baby ... complete in every way ... you will nurture them ... and protect them ... and love them ... so while I stay quiet for a while perhaps you would like to do this now ... just quietly in your head/imagination ... and then listen very attentively for their answer ... it may not be in words ... just in your senses ... but you will understand ... you and your precious little baby will understand each other perfectly.

The phrase 'it may not be in words' allows the woman to get a sense of an answer even if they cannot imagine actual words.

And you know that you can *return again and again to talk to your baby* so that you can really get to know each other ... you can create this special time for both of you where ... just like today ... you choose to sit down or lie down and *make yourself very comfortable* ... taking great care to ensure you are well supported ... allow your eyelids to close and *let your head sink back into the cushion/pillow* and *allow all the muscles to relax* ... relaxing the muscles in your shoulders ... and notice ... as you do so ... how *your shoulders seem to sink gently down into your arms* ... now *letting the arms relax so that any possible tension drifts down through your elbows ... down through your wrists ... down through your hands and out through your fingertips* ... finding just enough energy to let your hands gently rest on your stomach/abdomen ... just finding the most comfortable position for you and ... of course ... do know, that if you want to shift your position at any time to *increase your comfort* ... you will *do this naturally and easily* ... and I don't know whether you will *experience this as a* single wonderful *wave of comfort that flows all over your body or whether it will seem more like little ripples of comfort easing their way all down and all the way through your body* ... but you can *allow it to happen in just the right way for you* ... in just the right way for your baby ... and as you do this you will *remember the comfortable feelings in your body that you are feeling right now.*

Repeating the light relaxation induction serves a dual role. It reminds the client of the procedure to carry out at home and it also further deepens the current light trance state, increasing receptivity to the forthcoming suggestions

Reinforces and installs subsequent revivification of the feelings of trance

And as you become aware once again of the pure shining light and breathe it inside … you will also be reminded of just *how delightful it is and how easy it is* to *feel the connection with this little person inside you … see that image again in your mind's eye … clearly sensing the details of your baby's body … noticing perhaps how they've grown … how they've developed … delighting in how beautiful they are … and you will find that you become very creative in the ways that you can send love to your baby …* sending wave after wave of your love … sometimes very simply just through your breathing … you just *breathe that wonderful feeling of love through to your baby* and they will receive it … and they will *feel loved and cherished.*

There are many ways to express love and this suggestion for creativity allows the client to do this in the most appropriate way for her

At other times you may *become aware of the beating of your heart* and you can *let your baby know that each gentle heartbeat is pulsing love from you to them* … they will be reassured and comforted by that regular, gentle, beat of your love … and of course the comfort of your heartbeat will reassure them all night long even as you sleep.

The heart has long been considered the seat of love. It is a particularly useful metaphor as the physical beating of the heart continues day and night

And sometimes you will want to *talk/chat to your baby in a very natural way* … perhaps giving them news about what you've been doing or telling them about your preparations for their arrival … telling them how excited you are … and always making time to listen to how they are … what they need from you … really enjoying your special time together … taking that time for both of you to *feel so at ease … so at home with one another* … so that when the time comes for Baby's birth it will be the happiest and the most natural and comfortable meeting in the world.

Communication can just be in the manner of everyday 'chit chat'

Seeds the idea of an easy, happy birth

And taking a few more moments now to enjoy this pleasant, gentle state of relaxation … so nice for you both … it's good to realize that even staying very lightly relaxed … just drifting and dreaming … your unconscious mind can *absorb powerful suggestions for your good health, a positive outlook and a sense of contentment that will have profound effects on your frame of mind and on your physical well-being* ... your mind and your body are in perfect harmony ... every night as you sleep *your body replenishes its stores of energy ... you sleep well ... really well* ... and when you wake in the morning *you feel well rested and experience a sense of well-being and enthusiasm for the day ahead* ... and over the next few weeks it may surprise you to *notice how well you feel* ... and people will be commenting on *how well you look.* (Of course you're always going to come across those strange but well-meaning people from time to time who think they are showing their friendship or concern for you by asking you if you're feeling tired or unwell but you will find yourself laughing and replying ... 'No, *I feel* marvellous ... I have all the energy I need and I'm really enjoying this pregnancy.' Can you hear your voice? '*I feel* marvellous ... I have all the energy I need and I'm really enjoying this pregnancy.')

Primes the mind to accept the positive suggestions for mental and physical well-being which follow

Anchors a positive suggestion to counter possible thoughtless remarks made by unthinking friends and acquaintances

And the fact is that you really will *find yourself enjoying your pregnancy* ... understanding that you will pass through several stages which are normal and natural as well as being quite amazing! You may find yourself full of wonder at how your body knows instinctively how to *nurture your baby* and *take care of your own health and well-being* at the same time.

Embedded command to take care of their health

Go to a suitable trance reorientation or incorporate appropriate suggestions from one of the following short scripts before doing so

Anticipate positive childbirth (change beliefs)

What wonderful news ... you're going to have a baby ... I'm so pleased for you ... and I suppose it's natural that you might be wondering how it's going to *be (easy)* and how *you're going to feel (fine)* ... and you mentioned earlier that you had some vague anxieties about the birth ... partly because misguided people have told unhelpful stories ... strange, isn't it, how some people like to exaggerate stories for five minutes of fame? ... The truth is ... when you *stop and really think about it (confidently)*... that women have been giving birth for thousands of years and our bodies have this innate knowledge and ability to *do this naturally and easily* ... we may not necessarily know consciously exactly how it's done but *it's safe* (to give birth) to say that our bodies *do just know how to do it with consummate ease(ily) drift deeper into this relaxed state now* ... deeper and deeper where you can safely let any scary thoughts ... feelings ... images or words that had stuck in your mind from stories people had told ... even from long, long ago ... drift up from the darker recesses of your mind to the brighter surface where *you can see them in a completely different light* ... you know how it is ... when half-truths and mistaken and misleading ideas lurk in the shadows of your mind it can be a bit tricky/difficult to *see through them for the frauds they really are* but ... when you let them see the light of day ... *everything can seem so (safely) different.*

So as you allow any unhelpful thoughts, feelings or images to *float up to the surface now* ... you can let them float over there onto that board ... maybe it's a blackboard or perhaps it's a white board or possibly even one of those amazing magic boards linked to a computer ... and *look at those worries honestly* ... and *with your new understanding* ... expose the simply scaremongering stories/old wives' tales ... perhaps understand the motives of other people's

A useful strategy in hypnotic intervention is to intersperse positive words in your suggestions that may or may not necessarily make perfect, *or indeed any*, grammatical sense but can be picked up at the unconscious level. In addition, a word may be placed at the end of one phrase but also serve to introduce the next. This is intentionally confusing for the client's conscious mind. (Where I have used either of the above devices I have placed the words in brackets.) If you prefer a script to be totally clear and straightforward you can of course omit the confusing insertions

A liberal scattering of the words 'safe' and 'safely' anywhere in the script is useful as it will help to form the unconscious link between birth and safety

Pre-supposition that there is a 'new understanding'

exaggerations … maybe now … with the surprisingly sudden maturity and strength that pregnancy confers …*you will find that the effect of what you had been thinking previously has lessened* … even *disappeared already* … but take a look at anything unwanted that has remained and calmly pick up your eraser and rub it off the board … or if you have one of those magic boards, all you need to do is to touch the offending words or images and they will just disappear … that's it … *erase all the old stuff* and now *write up new positive beliefs in strong bright colours* … My body has a natural and innate ability to *give birth easily* … my body knows what to do at the unconscious level … I give myself permission to *experience this birth in a positive way* … I will *have all the energy and focus I need* … I give myself the permission to *enjoy my entire pregnancy* and I'm looking forward to meeting my lovely/precious/adorable/so-much-wanted baby for the first time at the birth … well done. Now, if *you want to, add in any other positive beliefs that will stay with you and sustain you throughout your entire pregnancy and throughout your baby's birth* (will be a positive experience).

Presupposition that there is a 'surprisingly sudden maturity'

Leave sufficiently long pauses for them to mentally write up the suggestions on their internal board

Well done … take a moment or two to read through those positive new beliefs once more … and take a deep breath as you read each one … and each one will be breathed deep inside and *become a very real part of your deep inner mind* … *become a very real part of your deep inner way of thinking positively* … *become a very real part of your deep inner way of feeling calm* … that's right … safely inside you (are amazing).

Go to a suitable reorientation or a further script

Preparing to give birth – installing positive anchors

Very soon now it will be time for your baby to be born … how very exciting … are you wondering just what it will be like to hold this precious little bundle/ this tiny little being/this beautiful little baby in your arms and know that this is your very own child … this is the little person you've been nurturing inside you for all these months and now you can actually hold him or her in your arms at last … how wonder-ful it's going to be … what an amazing experience this is going to be … and, of course, *you* already know … because you've chosen to come to see me today … how *the power of your unconscious mind can influence your conscious mind and your body in the very best of ways* … you know how your unconscious mind can direct your conscious mind to *stay confident and calm wherever you are … whenever you're there … whatever you're doing and whomever you're with* … and not only that … your unconscious mind can direct your body to create the very best of experiences so that *giving birth to your baby will be a wonderful experience* … and as you *drift deeper into the relaxed state*, we're going to create a link with the palm of your hand to *powerful inner resources that will support and sustain you as you go through every stage of birth.*

So now … let the sound of my voice relax you even further … hearing and feeling my voice taking you deeper and deeper into the pleasant yet power-ful trance state where *your mind and body work together in perfect harmony* … let each in breath fill you with calm … and let each out breath *release any possible tension* … release any possible ten-sion in your mind … release any possible tension in your body … and as you *drift deeper and deeper into this comfortable state of ease and relaxation* … you'll find that each out breath increases this sense of easy calm and you can begin to *notice the sense of mind and body harmony developing more and more within you* … every part of you in touch … one

Initial focus is on the arrival of the baby rather than on the process of birth

Reassuring to let people know what you are going to do

Reminder that the state is not only pleasant but also powerful with the other ... your easy natural breathing simply increasing those feelings of positivity in your mind and naturally bringing to mind occasions/times in your life where you have felt very positive ... times where you have been very determined ... times where you have been aware of the strength within you ... times where you have been aware of an inner energy ... times where you have experienced a sense of excitement ... and ... as you begin to *become more and more aware of those feelings inside* ... I'd like you to press your thumb firmly into the palm of your other hand and move it gently around and around ... *reawakening and strengthening those feelings* ... and say to yourself ... 'I am strong ... I am calm ... I am determined ... I have all the energy I need' and then notice how your mind is delving even deeper into all your inner reserves and reinforcing those resources ... making them available to you now ... feel them ... all the while moving your thumb round and around in your palm while you say again to yourself 'I am strong ... I am calm ... I am determined ... I have all the energy I need' ... and all the while you have been becoming more and more receptive in your mind to those suggestions you want and need to hear ... they are embedding themselves strongly inside you.

And it's so good to know *you have all the mental and physical and emotional reserves and resources you need for a successful/an easy birth* ... whenever you want to *be even more aware of these internal resources,* you will place your thumb in the palm of your other hand and you will seem to *hear my voice saying to you* ... this is exciting ... you are strong ... you are calm ... and you will repeat that to yourself mentally ... 'this is exciting ... I am strong ... I am calm' ... and you will also hear my voice telling you ... you are determined ... that's it, repeat it mentally ... 'I am determined' ... you have all the energy you need ... that's right, repeat it mentally ... 'I have all the energy I need'. ... Well done/Great job ... so whenever you want to feel an extra boost of these

Links breathing with positive experiences

Also include specific positive experiences elicited in your pre-trance discussion

Installing a physical anchor

Increasing the strength of the anchor verbally

Presupposition that the inner resources exist

Presupposes that inner resources for an easy birth exist. This suggestion is then linked to the previously installed physical anchor

'Exciting' is a good reframe of anxiety

Asking the client to repeat the words mentally not only provides repetition of the suggestions but also increases the power of the words through 'I' statements

resources, simply move your thumb around the palm of your other hand and it will bring back these wonderful feelings that you are feeling right now … and what's more … if for whatever reason you couldn't actually make the physical gesture … *you can simply imagine doing it and all those positive feelings will come back into your body* … go on now … let your hands part and now just imagine putting your thumb into your palm and moving it around … now hear that inner voice reassuring you … repeat the words to yourself … and just *feel how good you feel right now* … great.

It is useful to practise doing this merely in the imagination since there may be practical reasons why it cannot be done during the actual birth

So, at any time before or during the birth … any time you want an extra boost of positive energy and confident calm … this is exactly what you do … you touch the palm of your hand … just as you've done before … and stir up those great feelings … so let's just take a moment or two right now to see just how *you can make use of this for the birth* … imagine you can see yourself in hospital/at home when you want/need a boost of confidence and calm … see yourself just touching your thumb to your palm and moving it around … see how well you respond … *notice yourself hearing the inner voice instilling positive feelings … feel the boost of energy* … how exciting … you will soon be meeting your baby.

Reinforces the positivity anchor

Positive visualisation of the anchor in use

VAK

Take a look at yourself handling everything so well … see how *the moment you become aware of a sensation within* that lets you know Baby is on his or her way … you can touch your thumb to your palm … move it around and *you will receive a boost of confidence … a surge of energy and positivity … that 'Yes, I can' feeling* that some women describe as being like the excitement of surfing along the crest of a wave … and these waves are all … of course … part of the process that allows the *birth canal to open wider so your baby can travel along with ease* … and as *you* get this wave of energy and confidence … you might like to transmit the same message to *your baby* … 'I can do this and you can

More visualisation and more reinforcement of the positivity anchor

Introduces the analogy of the excitement of surfing along the waves

Mentally talking to and encouraging the baby on the journey can increase the sense of togetherness

do this too … we can do it together … I'm so excited I'm going to hold you in my arms soon' … look at yourself there … *you have all the resources you need* and it's interesting to see how *you somehow manage to be calm and excited at the same time* … and sometimes the waves are higher or stronger and just pressing your thumb into your palm allows you to ride along the waves until they tumble over into white surf as they *subside and you take a rest and breathe … breathe out the tension and breathe in the calm* and know your baby is coming ever closer and closer … well done.

The metaphor of the wave allows reframing of pain

Embedded command

And no doubt you will be thinking how pleased you are that *you have a powerful trigger in your palm for calm and confidence and energy whenever you need it* … in fact, now the palm of your hand is so strongly connected to those positive feelings … *you will find a surge of positivity comes over you at any time during the birth … even when you just hold/ grasp someone's hand* … just holding the hand of your husband/your partner/your midwife/a nurse/a doctor … or even simply holding the bedclothes … will *trigger that wonderful surge of positivity and you will have that 'Yes, I can do this' feeling.*

A natural instinct during a contraction may be to grasp someone's hand so this section links this action to the same positive feelings as before

You can include time distortion suggestions as given in the *Speed up or slow down time during labour* script

Add in any other appropriate suggestions and follow by ego strengthening and a suitable trance reorientation

Speed up or slow down time during labour

These suggestions are also used in the *Take care of your health* script but are reproduced separately here so that they may be used independently or in conjunction with a different script.

Interesting how *your mind can affect your body in such a positive way* … you know how it is when we are busy or absorbed in thought … we can *completely ignore minor aches and pains* because *we are focused on something else entirely* … there is a part of your mind which instinctively knows when to pay attention and when *not* to pay attention to particular sensations or thoughts … and when that part knows that *certain sensations or thoughts are of no significance at all* … it can choose to *let them wash over you as of absolutely no significance at all … hardly aware of them at all* … and that part is much the same part that lets your mind *experience time in different ways* … the time waiting for a bus in the rain may be exactly the same *clock* time as the time spent writing an email/reading a book/talking to your best friend on the telephone or getting ready to go out when you're already late … but we all know which *time seems to go faster* … so we already have the natural ability to *speed up or slow down our perception of time at the unconscious level* and now … in this hypnotic state … using hypnotic thinking … you can *strengthen that unconscious ability to perceive time differently* whenever you need to … whenever you want to … and so during the birth you will discover that the *time with contractions will speed up … will pass more quickly* … will *seem fairly brief/easily bearable* … for, of course, in the totality of your life … in the totality of your pregnancy … this time is nothing at all … while time between the waves when *you feel well rested, calm and you are re-energising will slow down* and you can really *enjoy those calm comfortable feelings* for so much longer … and *you tend to be very aware of that time when you're recouping your energy … feeling almost buoyant* … you *notice how positive you feel … and*

> **Seeds the idea of time or sensations being perceived differently according to our focus of attention**

> **Suggests that the ability to speed up or slow down perceived time is natural and that this ability can be enhanced through the hypnotic state**

191

those people around you ... the midwives ... your husband/partner/the doctor seem to *notice and comment on how good you look ... how well you are handling the situation.*

So why not take a little time now ... which might seem like a long time ... *to see yourself in your mind's eye, how things are going so well during labour and the birth* ... look at how you are dealing with everything so well as you are so focused on the fact that your precious baby will soon be here ... your mind has learned its lesson very well without even consciously thinking how it managed it ... *it's speeding up any possible down time so you are coping with it easily and calmly ... you can bear any waves of sensations with great equanimity because you know they will pass quickly ... that's right ... your unconscious mind is reminding you that with each wave you are helping your baby along their journey, you are making their journey easier so you can derive a great deal of satisfaction from that ... and your mind will also do something else amazing ... it will slow down every minute of comfortable, positive time so you can* relish the feeling and the knowledge that your baby will soon be with you ... (what a wonderfully exciting time this is!) ... and when you look back after the birth ... and you will do ... you will know that you *were able to take everything in your stride at this very special time.*

Add in specific suggestions relevant to their situation. Get them to visualise carrying out their desired outcome calmly and confidently

Go to a suitable trance reorientation or add in further appropriate suggestions

Rapid healing after childbirth

In order to avoid clumsiness in the script I have referred to a baby son and used masculine pronouns throughout.

So now you have given birth to your lovely son, (William) (and can hold him in your arms) … how wonderful … you have already begun the amazing experience of learning from each other and growing together … growing stronger … growing closer … growing more experienced together … and this will continue every day … sometimes surprising each other and sometimes feeling just so familiar with each other that it feels as though you have been doing it for a life time as you and (William) are learning from each other … a most amazing team.

Omit 'can hold him in your arms' **if this is not appropriate**

Using the baby's name creates good rapport and encourages bonding

All of your body's natural healing forces are also coming into play … and in this state of deep relaxation and light hypnotic trance … feeling so calm as you listen to the sound of my voice … isn't it good to know that your unconscious mind can encourage rapid healing and enhance the recovery process and, of course, it's reassuring to *remember that these simple natural processes in the body are continually working for us outside our conscious awareness* … we don't normally *notice all the times when our skin heals cuts and grazes all on its own* … we just *accept that this is what happens naturally* and, of course, it *does* happen naturally and has done so countless times in your lifetime and I wonder how … right now … *you can enhance that healing process* by imagining … in whatever way is right for you … this process occurring … maybe you can *see it in your mind's eye* as a gentle beam of golden light that soothes as it heals every place it is directed on your body … maybe *you are even becoming aware of this healing taking place right now* … your skin repairing and renewing throughout every layer … and now the light shining through even more deeply and healing

'I wonder **how**' rather than 'I wonder **if**' presupposes that the healing process can be enhanced

V and K imagery

internally too ... possibly with a sense of warmth or gentle tingling letting you know that it is indeed happening right now? [Pause]

Positive reframing of any possible sore or smarting sensations as tingling or warmth

And now imagine a light mist of soothing balm ... that you could step into so that it caresses your body ... a balm that has healing emollients that smooth into your skin ... that soothe you and calm you as the mist cools you a little now ... a mist that is so fine and gentle that you can only just feel it stroking you as it performs its miracle ... helping the skin to heal over ... encouraging skin cells to renew themselves ... wonderful, enhanced, rapid healing. [Pause] Now you have given birth to your amazing baby, (William), your body knows just what it needs to do naturally and easily ... all the pregnancy hormones understand they have done their very best and know their work is done now ... they are receding at just the right rate and in just the right way to bring the greatest comfort and the greatest ease to your body all over and all the way through ... all the tissues and all the muscles in your body are ready to move on ... they are ready to regain their shape ... regain their tone ... your body is naturally eager to firm up ... to feel that vitality once again ... perhaps you can even become aware of an inner stirring ... a readiness to move forward to the next stage ... the healing and recuperation will happen naturally ... you *speed up the process as you see it ... feel it ... experience it with all the senses* ... a sense of strength ... yes, everyday a little stronger ... a little more energised ... reinvigorated.

V and K imagery now invoking a cooling effect

Suggestions for healing the skin will be particularly appropriate where there has been an episiotomy or caesarean section. You can elaborate further if necessary with more words of healing and renewal

You will find that your body continues to renew, regenerate and recover as you rest ... not only while you sleep ... *rest and sleep surprisingly well* ... and life can be full of surprises ... and I wonder if you will *surprise yourself how well you cope over the next few days and weeks* ... how you take every little opportunity to rest and how you can *feel quite rested even with less sleep* than before ... and who, I'm wondering, will be most delighted ... you or your

A suggestion for recovery *while resting* is useful since actual sleep may be in short supply initially (despite a suggestion for sleeping well)

midwife/medical team *when they tell you how well
you are recovering … 'You are doing so well … what
excellent progress.' And not only are you coping well
physically … you are feeling positive and optimistic
too … enjoying being with your baby and enjoying
being a mum/mother (all over again).*   Include *'all over again'* **if this
is not a first baby**

Go to a suitable trance reorientation or add further suggestions from the following notes

Variations, Adaptations and Recommendations

Other suitable scripts, either in their entirety or selected extracts, would include *Recovery from surgery* or some of those to be found in the *Coping with Pain* section. *Mother and baby teamwork* will be useful to help bonding with the baby and for increasing or decreasing the flow of breast milk. Be attentive in your pre-trance discussion to any signs of post-natal depression and adjust scripts accordingly. Recommend discussing it with a physician if you have serious concerns. In the case of early signs of post-natal depression, you could also look at the scripts in the section on *Mild to Moderate Depression* and adapt those to the individual circumstances of your client.

Mother and baby teamwork – caring for and feeding your baby

In order to avoid clumsiness in the script I have referred to a baby daughter and used feminine pronouns throughout.

The script offers options regarding stimulating or inhibiting milk production according to breast or bottle feeding. Read through and choose the appropriate version for your client.

So now you have given birth to your lovely daughter, Maddie (and can hold her in your arms) ... how wonderful ... you have already begun the amazing experience of learning from each other and growing together ... growing stronger ... growing closer ... growing more experienced together ... and this will continue every day ... sometimes surprising each other and sometimes feeling just so familiar with each other that it feels as though you have been doing it for a lifetime ... (and, of course, you have indeed been nurturing and loving (Maddie) all of her little life from the very beginning).

Omit 'can hold her in your arms' **if this is not appropriate**

Using the baby's name can help bonding right from the start but in case of any 'sudden onset therapist amnesia' for the gender or the name, I believe it always sounds appropriate to just say 'Baby'!

Every day now is full of learning experiences ... you, learning how best to *hold her and support her* ... both of you learning together how to *feed easily* ... you, finding out her likes and her dislikes ... she, discovering how to interact with her new environment ... and when you *stop ... and think about it* ... this is really how life is ... (is it not?) ... in so many aspects ... we live and we experience and we learn things together and this can be one of the very best ways of learning ... certainly one of the most enjoyable ways of learning ... taking advice where and when and from whom appropriate ... but learning to *trust your own instincts too* as you gain more and more experience ... using your eyes ... your ears ... your touch ... your mind and, of course, your intuition as you *gain more and more confidence too.*

Truism

So as you and Baby (and Dad) are learning from each other ... a most amazing team ... (you are all

Omit 'Dad' **and the reference to** 'being a family together' **if not appropriate**

196

enjoying being a family together) … and all the while your body's natural healing forces are also coming into play … and in this state of deep relaxation and light hypnotic trance … feeling so calm as you listen to the sound of my voice … isn't it good to know that your unconscious mind can encourage rapid healing and enhance the recovery process and, of course, it's reassuring to *remember that these simple natural processes in the body are continually working for us outside our conscious awareness … this is what happens naturally* as you and your baby get on with learning more and more about each other … getting to know each other … you, becoming more and more accustomed to holding and supporting her in the way she likes best … enjoying the little routines of feeding and washing and changing her … making her more comfortable … and she is recognizing you by your touch … by your voice … by your smell … and you are so important to her … what a team … growing closer every day.

And you told me that you are breast feeding (Maddie) … how lovely … another opportunity for you to grow closer to each other as she nuzzles into you as she feeds … maybe you can take a moment or two now to capture this experience in your imagination for a moment because … as I mentioned before … in the process of hypnosis … your unconscious mind can enhance the simple natural processes of the body so that … not only are all the healing forces coming into play, but also all the natural processes of motherhood can be enhanced … seeing and feeling your baby feeding from you in your imagination right now … can help increase the production of milk … seeing in your mind's eye that *you have a more than ample supply* … feeling it flow easily and steadily as your baby feeds … she has all the nourishment she needs … she feels good and calm and you feel good and calm … the perfect team … and every day you can do this in your imagination if you want to stimulate the production and increase the flow … tell yourself … *I can produce all the milk my baby needs*

Breast feeding option

... it will flow easily, naturally and comfortably ... and now you can move her to your other side and use all of your senses again to enhance the process a little more ... see her contented little face, hear those satisfied little sounds as she feeds and feel the milk flowing easily and tell yourself you have all the milk she needs ... that's right ... that's completely right ... well done.

And you told me that you are bottle feeding (Maddie) ... so here and now in this lovely relaxing state of trance where your unconscious mind is so receptive to suggestion ... you can explain gently yet firmly to the part of you that runs/controls your body ... that you have no need of milk ... ask that part of you to stop the flow of milk/let the flow of milk gently but surely dry up since neither you nor your baby have any need of it at all ... thank it for any efforts it has made on your behalf to produce milk but explain that your baby has all the milk she needs ... she has all the nourishment she needs ... you are taking care of (Maddie) in a different way ... the milk can gently dry up in a very natural way ... that's right ... that's completely right ... well done ... now take a moment or two to visualise feeding (Maddie) with her bottle ... see how happy she is ... see how she has all the nourishment she needs and notice that your breasts have returned to normal ... your body understands that there is no need for milk ... you have no need for milk ... (Maddie) has all the milk she needs in her bottle and you are both very comfortable with that ... look at her in your arms ... see how happy she looks ... feel her contentment ... she's very well fed and you are very comfortable with that.

Bottle feeding option

Some mothers say that they feel (or are encouraged to feel) guilty for choosing not to breastfeed. These suggestions would help them to feel at ease with their decision

Go to a suitable trance reorientation or add further suggestions from the selection of scripts mentioned in the box below

Variations, Adaptations and Recommendations

Other suitable scripts, either in their entirety or selected extracts, would include *Rapid healing after childbirth, Recovery from surgery* or any of those to be found in the **Coping with Pain** section.

Enhance Business Performance

All the scripts in this section are suitable for use in a workplace coaching environment as well as in the hypnotherapy office/consulting room. If using them as a coaching tool, it may simply be appropriate to ask the client just to close their eyes and use their imagination with no obvious induction at all. If you do choose to use an induction however, I would suggest that you select one that is simple and light and appropriate for the office environment. *The Lift or elevator* or an adaptation of *'Yes set' questions and statements*, perhaps omitting reference to the hypnotic state, would be very suitable. In practice, when people become absorbed in inner contemplation and imaginative activity they are accessing light states, and sometimes deep states, of trance without the need for anything more formal at all.

Even when using the scripts in a typical hypnotherapy environment, I would still suggest a light state of trance is more than adequate for this type of work as it seems to work well with a blend of conscious and unconscious activity.

It is essential to read the scripts thoroughly before use since some of them offer options in the text, and some will work best when certain ideas are discussed in advance and others will be more effective if personal reference experiences can be elicited in discussion beforehand and alluded to in the script.

They are largely intended to be used in a 'content-free' manner so that the therapist avoids becoming over involved in the content and can use his or her skills to guide the client through the mental process itself, remembering to allow plenty of time for reflective thought. However, if it is more appropriate, they can all be adapted and used in a more interactive question and answer style.

Several metaphors such as 'downloading applications for fixing problems' or 'designing suits to protect against negativity or disappointment' have been used. If these are thought to be too complex or inappropriate in any way, I encourage you to use the underlying ideas and adapt the script in the way you see fit for your particular client.

Although they have been written with the workplace in mind, they could all easily be adapted, either in part or as a whole, for use in more personal contexts.

Goal/outcome setting – generic content-free script

This script has been designed to allow the client to complete the activity mentally and privately without actually talking about the content, although, if preferred, it can easily be adapted to make it interactive. One advantage of having the client perform it mentally is that the therapist doesn't get caught up in giving advice on the content but concerns him or herself with helping the client through the process. It is, of course, useful to explain this to the client and discuss general principles of goal setting beforehand. Emphasize the need for highly specific objectives stated in the positive. It is also useful to identify in advance motivational strategies which they have used successfully in the past.

Now … just sitting and making yourself comfortable … feeling the support of the chair … and letting yourself take a few minutes where you can take yourself off into your thoughts and develop a pleasant inner absorbed state where you can *see things from a different perspective* and where you can *be at your most creative* … so why not enjoy this experience as you set a goal/some goals that will improve the quality of your life? You told me that you are very sure that you both need and want to make some positive changes.

Very, very briefly now I'd like you to see a mental image of your future if things were to stay exactly how they are currently and if you were to change nothing at all … maybe see this on a mental computer screen … think about how things would be for you and for others … how you would feel … what you would be saying to yourself … what recriminations there might be. [Pause] Tell me or shake your head, No, when you are quite certain that this is definitely not what you want to happen. [Assuming a 'No'] Good decision.

Gives them an image of how life will be if no changes are made. In a moment they will compare this with an image of their desired outcome with all changes achieved. The aim is to increase motivation for change

So let's start with a very straightforward question for you to consider and let me know when you have an answer that you are sure of. Don't tell me the answer … just let me know when you have it … Ready? …

Decide what is it that you really want to achieve. Take a moment ... mentally, silently to go over it in your mind ... making quite sure that it is very specific and that you phrase this to yourself in the positive ... *not* what you *don't* want ... think about what you *do* want. Let me know when you're ready to proceed. [Pause for agreement] Right. Let's double-check ... you have a very clear aim in your mind of what you want to achieve ... the aim is very specific and it is phrased in the positive, is that so? ... Good.

Have them identify a specific positive outcome (You will have discussed the value of this in your pre-trance discussion)

Just think for a moment of how things will be once you have achieved this outcome ... (no need to tell me) ... and then get a mental image of this ... perhaps on a computer screen or on a big movie screen ... notice where and when this outcome will be achieved and the very specific effects that this will have on you. What does this achievement do for you? How does it feel inside? What effects does this have on specific other people? What differences do you notice? Notice too how other people respond towards you. How does that feel to you? Now think about how it might affect any other projects; are there any other implications? If there are any negative implications, consider whether this makes your goal unworkable or are you prepared in a moment or two to see how you can work around this? Let me know when you are still sure that this goal/outcome is what you really want. [Pause] Excellent.

Give plenty of pauses throughout this section that are long enough to find their internal answers to your questions

If you were to get a negative answer, they will need to modify their aim or develop a new one

Put on your cool, calm, objective head that you use when you see the overall picture of things very clearly and check that *this goal/outcome is very specific* ... not wishy-washy/fuzzy in any way ... and that *it's something that is realistically possible for you to achieve* ... and as you look at the picture/movie, ask yourself whether you need any practical help or practical resources of any kind ... and if so ... have a think about what steps you could take to acquire them ... for example ... do you need to do some research? Is there a helpful course? Do you need some new equipment? [Pause] Now, look inside

Evaluate the desired outcome

Visual

External practical resources

yourself and check on your own inner strengths and resources that will be useful to you in achieving this goal. [Pause] What help might you need perhaps from anybody else? Who can give you this help? [Pause] And I think you'll find it reassuring to know now ... that your unconscious mind has started a search which will continue in the background while you get on with your daily life ... and over the next few days *useful thoughts and ideas may just pop into your mind* when you least expect them ... and you will find yourself thinking 'Of course, that's it ... it all seems so obvious now.' ... So now it's time to move onto the next stage of putting some very specific steps in place and checking the necessary timings but ... just before we do ... quickly check out if there is any other aspect that you need to consider before we move on ... and nod your head when you're ready to move on. [Pause] Excellent.

Inner resources

Reassurance that the unconscious mind will continue searching for positive ideas over the next few days

Now is the time for you to consider the specific steps you need to put in place in order to ensure that everything happens just as you want it to do ... at the specific time that you want it to happen ... co-ordinating all help and resources as you go along ... thinking about how long any specific steps might take you. [Pause] Let me know once you've done that ... Good, now talk it over with the part of yourself that is good at handling problems/ troubleshooting and see whether you can come up with any specific advice to *ensure this project works exactly as you want it to*. [Pause] Is there any tip or strategy you have used successfully in the past that would be useful to include here?

Put time-specific steps in place

Presupposition that there is a 'part of yourself that is good at handling problems'

Use successful strategy from the past

So, all looking good, sounding good and feeling good inside ... I'd like you to have a look at that screen once more and see yourself running through every step of the way until *your outcome is achieved* and let me know once you've done it. [Pause] Good job ... now I invite you to *see it in a slightly different way* ... this time, starting at the end where you have already achieved your goal ... working backwards

VAK

Visualisation of success

to check everything was correctly in place when you needed it. [Pause] Excellent job … so just to make absolutely sure that you have considered this from every angle and got to grips with every detail … is there anything else at all that you want to include or to change so that *nothing can stand in the way of success*? If so, see it through again now from beginning to end and include that extra step. [Pause]

Kinaesthetic

So just before we finish, it is important to commit to all of this by recording it in some way … so I would like you to type that goal into your mental computer/ laptop … (or write it in a mental notebook) … make sure your goal is stated in the positive and make it very specific … look at it on the screen and check it's what you really want … highlight it in your chosen colour … and *save that information*.

Commit goals and outcomes to mental computer

Positive and specific

Now type in the benefits this achievement will get for you … both practical and emotional … look at them on the screen and check *these benefits are what you really want* … highlight them in your chosen colour … and *save that information.*

Benefits to you

Now add in the benefits to other people if there are others involved in any way … once more, check them on the screen and check that *you really want this* … highlight them in your chosen colour … and *save that information*.

Benefits to others

Type in any tip or useful strategy from the past and also any practical and emotional reward to motivate yourself if you were to need a bit of extra encouragement along the way … highlight them in your chosen colour … and *save that* information.

Motivation strategies from the past

Give them enough time to think of a reward

Type in each step with timings … check all resources are in place and now … as you save that information … take a moment or two to *step right into the process and zoom forward into the wonderful feeling of achievement* … feel the results … hear the results … see the results … all yours … great ... excellent

Associate into successful achievement

VAK

job! ... What is the most satisfying thing about your success, I wonder?

So you have your plan in place ... you've made some very useful/wise/practical decisions ... created some excellent plans and now it's almost time for you to reorient yourself to the present and to the room with me ... isn't it good to know that, not only have you used your conscious mind, but *your unconscious mind too will be supporting you every step of the way* ... your unconscious mind is powerful and will help you *carry out all these plans and suggestions long after this session is over* ... breaking down each task into smaller chunks as and when necessary ... *you are powerful and you like this feeling of forward movement and achievement ... you enjoy the sense of relief once you have made your decisions ... feel how satisfying it is to do what you know you have to do* ... the sense of achievement as you just get on with it ... notice how ... as you are already beginning to reorient ... there is a compulsion to get back and *commit all these things to paper or to a document on your computer* ... you *feel compelled to do whatever it is that you need to do to achieve your aim* ... you are already on the path and headed in the right direction ... nothing can stop you now ... congratulations ... well done ... what an achievement!

Encouragement and reinforcement

Conscious and unconscious minds working in harmony to give support

Suggestion to commit it all to paper/computer on return home or to the office

Go to a suitable energising trance reorientation

Learn to delegate

This script assumes that the person has the authority to delegate (he or she is probably a manager) but finds difficulty in doing so for one reason or another. Your pre-trance discussions will allow you to adapt the middle sections to suit your client. You may want to omit several sections if they are not relevant or you can personalise suggestions when they have spoken of specific changes they wish to make.

And now … briefly … I'd like you to think about the time that you will free up … what you will do with it? … How will that make a difference to your working life? … And perhaps to your home life too? … Consider the differences it will make to colleagues/customers/clients/productivity … imagine right now that *you have somehow managed to free up this time* and *really notice those advantages to you … hearing those inner thoughts of yours … seeing the detail as well as the bigger picture … becoming aware of any gut feelings … and realise just why reclaiming this time is so important to you and just how positive it's going to be from now on/here on in.* [Pause]

> **Personalise this section with appropriate references to their individual situation elicited in the pre-trance discussion**
>
> **VAK**
>
> **Give adequate time for reflection before moving on to the next section**

Now I suggest that you rerun in your mind some of those occasions at work/in the office where you were just overloaded with work … just have a look at the 'you' on your internal mental screen in a detached kind of way … and … being very focused indeed … check out which of those tasks that you are engaged in **could** be done by somebody else … which of them really **should** be done by somebody else so that you *free yourself up to do other tasks which are more deserving of your attention* … so you *do more of those so-called 'higher leverage' tasks* or projects from which you/your company can get real benefit. [Pause] No need to tell me what they are, just let me know once you have identified those tasks. [Pause] Good.

> **Give adequate time for refection before moving on to the next section**

And now take another close look on that internal screen at what you *used* to do and how you *used* to do it ... see yourself busying yourself with all those things that really could or should have been done by somebody else and consider ... and I mean *really* consider ... whether some of the factors I'm going to mention may have played a part in your old reluctance to delegate. For example, sometimes people use the excuse that delegation creates too much risk of mistakes being made ... they are being 'over' perfectionist ... whereas in fact the art is to *learn the process of effective delegation ... to teach staff well so that risk is minimised ... to put safeguards in place ... to set up systems that minimise risk ...* and of course this is part of a manager's real responsibility. Time you spend doing this now will be saved over and over and over again later.

Deliberate change of tense in 'what you used to do'

Other times people just love to be 'the expert' and relish the opportunity to 'show off' their skills and knowledge and can't seem to resist doing everything just to get that praise/acknowledgement for doing it so well, when really it would be far more sensible to *let others do it and free up your time* ... or some people really love to be helpful and end up taking on other people's responsibilities because they don't like to say 'No' ... Other times people actually enjoy a particular task so much that they want to keep it, because it's fun/easy/satisfying whereas *the truth is that far better use could be made of their time.*

Give plenty of pauses for consideration

Embedded command

Then there is the issue of insecurity ... sometimes people hold onto a job because they fear the competition ... they fear that others would shine and do it better once they learned how to do it ... or they fear being challenged ... so It's particularly useful to know how here ... in this slightly altered state of awareness ... you can *get in touch with your inner confidence resources* ... every confident feeling and thought stored in your unconscious mind over the years that you may have consciously forgotten about is stored there ... and can *begin to make itself*

A sense of insecurity often underlies a reluctance to delegate. The client may well recognise this when they hear your words and thus welcome the suggestions offered for confidence and self-belief

felt ... those strong, positive feelings can begin to flow into every part of you that requires a boost ... and as they do, while you continue to listen to the sound of my voice, you will begin to experience a deepening sense of belief in yourself ... an inner sense of security and self-worth that will make a real difference to the way you think, feel and do things from now on.

There is also the belief that 'it's quicker to do it myself than ask somebody else to do it' which of course is true *at first* but the trick is to *invest a little time and effort now to teach someone so well that you reap the benefit a little bit later* ... and *this benefit may come sooner than you think* ... how great when you never need do that task again because it has become somebody else's responsibility ... and with your good teaching they *learn the task well* ... and they can *learn to do it quickly* with the practice that you let them have.

Use your voice to embed commands to the client *'learn the task well'* **and** *'learn to do it quickly'* although ostensibly the phrases refer to others

Now sometimes a reason for lack of delegation is the belief that you can do a task better than anybody else ... and, of course, since you have been doing it for a very long time, it's almost certainly true to say that you probably can do it better than anyone else ... *right at this moment* ... but ... with *a bit of **your** good teaching and a bit of good practice* ... that other person may well *learn to do it quite effectively* too ... and you know ... when you *stop and really think about it* ... it's often also true to say that ... if they do the task adequately ... even though not as well as you ... doing the task adequately is in fact often quite good enough ... and the real benefit is that you have freed up your time to do something of greater value ... greater value to you ... greater value to your company ... (and possibly greater value to your family as well if it allows you more time to spend with them).

Now of course I wouldn't dream of saying which ... if any at all ... of these ... apply to you ... but you will *know the answer* better than anyone else ... because you know yourself better than anyone else ... so take a moment now ... being at your most honest and analytical ... to decide any behaviours that you need to change ... including any others you have observed in yourself that I didn't even think of mentioning ... and maybe ... as I just stay quiet for a little while ... you'll find that *you really enjoy planning the changes you will make to create maximum benefit to you and your workplace* ... even *get quite excited as you explore all kinds of possibilities* and you discover just how much *you really want to make those changes now* ... take all the time you need ... seeing different scenarios ... listening to your own voice explaining and teaching ... listening to and considering other people's ideas ... feeling a sense inside of the right way to do things ... and once you have been through just as much as you need to do in your mind at this particular time ... you can let me know ... being aware of course that now this process of change has begun ... it will *continue long after this session is finished both at the conscious and unconscious level.* [Pause]

Reassures the process will continue

Give them plenty of time before moving on

Well done ... and I want you to know that over the next few days ... and even while you sleep at night ... in addition to your conscious thought ... your unconscious mind will continue ... quite effortlessly ... to *find even more interesting changes to make* and also *find effective ways to implement these changes* ... the important thing is that it will happen at the perfect time for you ... you may find that suddenly an idea comes into your mind when you least expect it ... or you may wake in the morning and *an answer seems so completely obvious to you* that you can hardly believe you hadn't thought of it before ... sometimes you may surprise yourself by finding that *you are naturally implementing an effective delegation strategy to free up your time* ... just as though you have always done this since *it seems so perfectly natural … so perfectly sensible … so perfectly in tune with who you are and what you do.*

And later … as you reflect on how well you have been able to *carry out so many ideas* … I believe you will congratulate yourself for making those changes … congratulate yourself on how well you were able to *teach others* … how patient you were as both you and others learned to *take responsibilities and deal with things in a new and more effective way* … how systematic you have been in your approach … how you have learned to *find satisfaction in seeing others do things well because of the way you taught them* … and even how you were able to *accept that certain things can be done well enough* … although perhaps not exactly in the perfect way that you would have done them yourself … a realisation, in fact, that *you have all the inner resources you need … of strength, of determination, of insight to make these changes happen* … pleased and relieved, I believe, that your own skills are being put to greater use now and *you can derive a great deal of satisfaction through that.*

Asking them to look back from a future where these things have taken place also allows you to embed commands for present action

Include relevant personal suggestions

Go to a suitable, energising trance reorientation

211

Be resilient in the workplace

As you relax here a little more comfortably/deeply for a few moments I'd like you to reflect on the research carried out on the brain that has shown that when we *create a powerful image and go over and over it in our minds* ... that somehow ... at the unconscious level, without our ever needing to know consciously how it happens ... it creates an effect which is no longer merely in the imagination but *becomes our reality too* ... so I'm going to invite you to drift off in your imagination now to a place where you can *make full use of your creativity* to create an image that will *increase your resilience* in exactly the ways you want ... so this place may be somewhere that you always get your best ideas ... at your desk perhaps ... or walking around ... or at your computer ... or ... (who knows?) even in the bath, ... or it may simply *be somewhere deep inside yourself* where you can *become more aware of your own ability for creative thought* ... wherever it is, just *let yourself be there now* ... maybe remembering how it feels to dream up some original ideas and ... as you let that feeling develop ... perhaps you could consider a rather 'off the wall' idea.

> Explains the purpose of imaginative visualisation and so pre-empts any reluctance to engage. At the same time, use your voice to embed useful suggestions

> *'Considering'* an idea is easier to accept than being asked to carry it out

Let's imagine that you're going to design a special kind of suit for the workplace that will need to have some very special properties ... it will need to *be strong and yet very flexible* ... it will need to *have the resilience of rubber* ... it might remind you of a rubber ball ... a squash ball for example that will *bounce back powerfully time and time again* ... it will need to be protective yet light and easy to wear ... now here's the thing ... it will also need to be invisible so that nobody but you will be aware that you are wearing it ... easy to slip on and off whenever you want to *feel an extra bit of protective bounce* ... it will be completely non-absorbent so it will *shrug off any possible negativity* from any person, however irritating or difficult they may be ... or *shrug off any possible disappointment or frustration from* any event, no

> Use your voice to emphasize the various embedded commands

212

matter what it might be. … So take a few moments now to design your suit … adding in any essential properties … take some confidence and create a confident lining perhaps … think about how you're going to *make use of positive thinking* … could you create a very, very deep positive pocket perhaps? … So that … whenever you need some extra positivity … you just put your hand in your pocket and *feel that sense of optimism spreading into your hand and right through your whole being.*

Let's take a moment to create that optimistic and confident resource to keep in your pocket for easy access whenever you want it … just begin to rub your thumb and first couple of fingers gently together … and as you do … think back to a couple of very good decisions you've made and how well they turned out and *get a taste of that sense of satisfaction* … and now as you *keep gently rubbing those fingers and thumb together*, let your mind *turn to some of your best achievements* … that's it … with all the feelings of pride in yourself for your efforts … for your success … for your ability … remember how you arrived at the position you're in … the hard work … the wise decisions … maybe you can even hear in your head … 'you are the best candidate so you've got the job'/'you have really good ideas'/'you're the person we need'. And it's not only about what *you've already achieved* but what you *want to achieve* … what you are going to achieve … *feel those feelings of excitement inside as you get fired up with enthusiasm* … you're going to *make it happen* … yes, *you're going to make it happen* … and every time you want to *remember all this … really remember this and get fired up with enthusiasm all over again … you can put your hand into your pocket … real or in your imagination … and actively rub those fingers and thumb together and you will get this sense of excitement and eagerness all over again and so you can cope with any person … cope with any event … cope with any possible negativity and bounce back from any possible rejec-*

A question is a very useful form of suggestion

Select and omit suggestions as appropriate to your client.

Installation of confidence anchor. This will be even more effective if you personalise it by using their very own positive reference experiences elicited beforehand. If there has been bullying, you will need to look outside the workplace for confidence

Use your voice enthusiastically to inspire positivity

Reinforces the confidence anchor

tion or refusal ... you just get the feeling inside 'I'm going to make it happen' and so of course you do! So let your fingers relax now as we go on and you *continue building your resilience.*

And now you have your positive pocket and your flexible, resilient suit ... you could consider how and where you can add in other desirable resources ... where will you add in your sense of determination? Could it be woven into the fabric along with your belief in yourself? Add in any other properties you feel you need ... add any special design features that will ensure that ... as soon as you slip into this suit in the morning ... you will *feel an inner sense of outer protection* ... you will also *be aware of an inner strength and toughness* and you are able to *remain resilient and positive* ... no matter who you encounter during the day ... no matter what is going on around you ... *you know you can cope calmly and confidently* so that foolish words no longer bother or upset you ... they just bounce off so they don't disturb you at all ... *you believe in you ... you believe in who you are and you believe in what you do.*

Give the opportunity to add in more resources of their own choosing

Repetition 'in threes' is an effective device

Take a moment or two to run through in your mind any scenarios where you want to *be more resilient* ... Check that you have put on your 'resilience suit' and it's working at its optimum to protect you from any possible negativity from people's critical or even bullying comments and it's *keeping you buoyant* despite events having turned out in disappointing ways ... see how somehow you are able to *cope with it all with a firmness and resilience* that may even surprise you ... surprise and impress others too ... look at your easy, relaxed, self-assured body language ... *listen to your strong, confident and positive voice* ... hear your inner thoughts which are expressing determination and optimism ... if things don't go well, you find you are looking to see what is useful to *learn from a situation* so you can put it into practice on another occasion to *ensure a better result next time* ... you are able to *take responsibil-*

Personalise with information elicited in pre-trance discussion regarding desired outcomes

VAK

ity for your actions and ... if necessary ... you *take on board useful suggestions constructively* rather than dwell on criticism ... see, hear and *feel how positively you are dealing with things now* ... dealing with others ... dealing with yourself in a positive and optimistic way.

Great stuff ... remember how the research says that *the more often you do this in your mind, the more these confident responses will become second nature to you in your actual real-life situations* ... so *take two minutes every day to run through this positive visualisation in your mind's eye until there can be no question about it* ... *this is how you respond in your daily life optimistically* ... *confidently* ... *resiliently* ... well done.

Reminder of the value of continued positive visualisation

Go to a suitable energising trance reorientation

Procrastination: common reasons

Reasons listed in self-help books include:

- Feeling daunted by a task: it is too big, complex or overwhelming.
- Avoiding unpleasant/boring tasks; thinking that you 'don't feel like doing it'.
- Dithering over unimportant decisions which will make no difference to an outcome.
- Being overwhelmed by complex decisions so not starting them.
- Leaving things till the last minute, claiming to work better under pressure of a deadline.
- Being easily sidetracked.
- Doing all the short easy tasks first for instant satisfaction and shelving important ones.
- Finding it difficult to say no to requests for help, even if they are unreasonable or unnecessary.

The following script *Procrastination* offers some helpful suggestions to counteract some of these problems. Of course, as always, it is essential to discuss with your client what they see as causes and solutions to their problems and not to impose the solutions given here.

The script gives a framework and the *List of applications* which follows it is for you to select from as appropriate to the needs of your client. Limit the number used or it will be overwhelming. Of course, you can adapt the framework, ignore the list and use any other preferred appropriate suggestions.

Procrastination

This script uses a metaphor of an internal mental computer or phone which can download various applications to fix problems. This will likely only appeal to people who regularly use such equipment. A list of applications which fix various procrastination problems follows the script and these could be discussed with your client when you are eliciting their problems and discussing aims and objectives. Clearly, if there is no suitable solution on the list, you need to adapt and extemporise according to your client's needs.

Bear in mind that the *Wisdom Wizard* is a good catch-all solution.

Use a simple light induction.

So now you are feeling pleasantly and lightly relaxed you can reflect a little more on our earlier discussion where you told me about the various problems that you have been encountering because of your habit of regularly putting things off ... and because being in a light trance state/a state of hypnotic focus allows us to *be more creative ... be more observant and be more detached from a problem too* ... it is an ideal state for you to *see things from a different perspective and come up with some creative and effective solutions* ... so I would like that part of *you that is so good at identifying problems and finding solutions to come forward now and do a bit of interesting work ... that can be done all at the unconscious level.*

Restates problem

Seeds the idea of the hypnotic state inducing creativity and more detached observation from a different perspective

Presupposes a part exists that is good at finding solutions

So ... being creative right now ... imagine that you have an inner/internal PC/laptop/phone and have a look on the screen and rerun some of those occasions where you put off doing something that was really important ... just have a look at the 'you' on the screen in a detached kind of way ... and ... *really notice* what is stopping you from getting down to things ... and while you check those things out ... *hearing those inner thoughts ... seeing the detail as well as the bigger picture ... becoming aware of any gut reactions* ... please double-check and

VAK

217

let me know that you still believe that the two main problems are <u>finding complex tasks overwhelming</u> and <u>avoiding tasks that you simply don't like very much</u>. [Pause] Thank you ... and once again please double-check that you are really sure that you need and want to *make the changes* to enable you to *get down to things straight away and get on with things even if you don't much like the task ... Great.*

Adapt according to your client's needs

Remember that here in this absorbed state your unconscious mind is particularly open and receptive ... it will *take on all the ideas and suggestions that are right for you and will not only improve the quality of your work but give you a wonderful feeling of personal satisfaction too* ... just go to your mental PC/laptop/phone once again and click on the web connection where you can download exactly the application you need to solve your problem(s). Let's double-check the procedure ... first you need to look for the application <u>Chunk Down</u> in order to get to grips with complex problems ... find the icon and click on it and it will download the solution right now. Great ... then you save it, so that your application will run automatically from now on. Done it? Excellent. Now do the same thing with the icon called <u>Teeth gritter</u> which is the application that will help you get on with any task ... like it or not ... your unconscious mind will understand exactly how to do this without your conscious mind needing to know how it's done ... you will just be aware that your attitude is changing day by day and things are getting done because you *make them get done ... you have this inner conviction that you are up to the challenge ... you are actively enjoying the challenge.*

Select appropriate application from the list which follows the script

Select appropriate application from the list which follows the script

This <u>Chunk down</u> application is great ... with this application running perfectly you will have a far more positive attitude towards tasks ... you will find that those old overwhelmed feelings have turned into positive proactive thoughts as you *set aside the time to plan out the task and write down the plan* ... you will automatically find yourself working through these questions in your mind … how can I *break up this piece of work into manageable sized chunks/* tasks/substeps? … Where will I *keep the list of separate tasks that make up the whole* … will it be on my PC or will it be in a diary? Which way do I get most pleasure as I check them off on completion? How long will each one take? … Which can I fit into an hour? Are there any I can do on the train? Are there any 'bite sized' tasks I can have on my desk ready to attend to while I wait to be put through on phone calls, for example file a document, proofread a page? Are there any that can be delegated? It begins to seem more manageable now … does it not? … with your <u>chunk down</u> application installed … this is how you work now quite automatically … breaking down each large piece of work into smaller chunks as and when necessary and you work your way through every task until it is completed … *continue through every task until the whole project is completed* … good job!

<u>Teeth gritter</u> is brilliant … it just helps you come to the conclusion that there are indeed some tasks that you don't really *feel like doing* now … but suddenly you actually realise that you were never going to *feel like doing them* later either … you *stop kidding/fooling/deceiving yourself …* you simply grit your teeth and you get down to the task(s) … you break them down into smaller tasks if you want to … but you get on with them … you start them … you continue them and you finish them … and the best thing of all is that you get this wonderful sense of satisfaction while you are doing them … even the merest hint of an internal voice saying 'I don't feel like doing this' only serves to increase your determination to … *do it now and finish it now* … nothing will stop you now … nothing will get in your way … what a tremendous feeling of satisfaction!

Excellent ... so the last thing to do is to click on the programme with the image of you on screen with your new application(s) running perfectly so you can observe how *you have fixed the problem* so well ... your unconscious mind is supporting you every step of the way ... you get a strong sense of achievement ... look at you ... you look calm ... you seem very much in control ... listen, can you hear it in your voice? ... *You are powerful and you like this feeling of forward movement and achievement ... feel how satisfying it is to do what you know you have to do* ... the relief and sense of achievement as *you just get on with it ... everything happening on time and in time* ... some tasks inevitably you enjoy more than others ... that's life ... but the most important thing to you now is that liking the task seems secondary to getting on with it and getting it done ... for that is where *you are deriving your greatest sense of satisfaction* ... excellent job. ... Notice also the positive effect on your colleagues ... they seem to be giving you more co-operation and respect just as *you have a greater sense of self-respect too* ... you *feel compelled to do whatever it takes to achieve your aim* ... nothing can stop you now ... congratulations on what you have achieved here today ... you've made some very useful decisions ... you've made some excellent plans ... and your unconscious mind will work in harmony with your conscious mind to ensure that you carry every one of them out ... well done ... what an achievement!

Go to a suitable energising trance reorientation

This guided visualisation is content-free so it is suitable to 'future pace' any of the suggested solutions on the list with the presupposition that the desired changes have been made

220

List of applications for solving procrastination problems

Select as appropriate to your client.

Simple decision maker

Once this application is in place you find that you realise it is far easier than you used to think ... just *stop dithering and make the decision quickly and stick to it* ... don't question it again ... once you've made it ... just *make the decision work* ... understand that there is rarely only one way to do something ... you've made a decision so now make it work for you ... in fact you find that you *like the idea of training yourself to make quick decisions* in situations where the result isn't remotely crucial ... you find you *enjoy giving yourself little decisions to make as quickly as you can* and you stick to them so you *get into the habit of quick decision making* ... blue or black pen today? Walk on this side of the road or that one? Fish or meat? Make this phone call or that one?

This 'application' is appropriate for people who dither and put off simple, somewhat trivial decisions. It is for those who waste time agonising over decisions which basically won't make too much difference either way

NB This is NOT for important, complex decisions

Difficult or complex decision maker

Once this application is in place you will find yourself drawn to starting the process of decision ... this will not be taken lightly ... you first set a deadline for the decision to be made ... consider sharing this deadline with others ... then you start your research ... you collect all relevant information available ... you consult other experts/colleagues as appropriate ... you make a list of options and the consequences of each ... advantages and disadvantages ... you feel compelled to type them into a document or write them down ... each and every one ... it is impossible to resist ... you are logical ... you are able to take a step back and feel far more detached now as you consider the arguments ... you see things clearly and rationally ... making use of all your conscious and unconscious skills, knowledge and resources ... then before your deadline arrives ... you decide to make the decision ... with all that information, you make it wisely and you type your decision into

This 'application' is for people who tend to put off making a decision, or even thinking about it, because they don't like doing it or they think the process is too complex or difficult. The outcome of this type of procrastination is that eventually the time arrives for the decision to be taken and it is made hastily without sufficient thought or understanding of likely consequences

a document/write it down … (if it is really a major decision you may even choose to 'sleep on it' allowing your unconscious mind to know if it 'feels right' in the morning) … then you act on it knowing you have given this all the attention it deserved and now is the time for you to do it and move forward … you know what to do … you have a compulsion to do it … and you do it … excellent … congratulate yourself on your new strategy.

Chunk down

This application is great … now it's running perfectly you will have a far more positive attitude towards tasks … you will find that those old overwhelmed feelings have turned into positive proactive thoughts as you *set aside the time to plan out the task and write down the plan* … you will automatically find yourself working through these questions in your mind … how can I *break up this piece of work into manageable sized chunks*/tasks/substeps? … Where will I *keep the list of separate tasks that make up the whole* … will it be on my PC or will it be in a diary? Which way do I get most pleasure as I check them off on completion? How long will each one take? … Which can I fit into an hour? Are there any I can do on the train? Are there any 'bite sized' tasks I can have on my desk ready to attend to while I wait to be put through on phone calls, for example file a document, proofread a page? Are there any that can be delegated? It begins to seem more manageable now … does it not? … with your <u>chunk down</u> application installed … this is how you work now quite automatically … breaking down each large piece of work into smaller chunks as and when necessary and you work your way through every task until it is completed … *continue through every task until the whole project is completed* … good job!

This 'application' is for people who tend to feel overwhelmed by the size or complexity of the task

Teeth gritter

This application is brilliant … it just helps you come to the conclusion that there are indeed some tasks that you don't really *feel like doing* now … but

This 'application' is for people who don't like the task and simply need to grit their teeth and do it

suddenly you actually realise that you were never going to *feel like doing them* later either … you *stop kidding/fooling/deceiving yourself* … you simply grit your teeth and you get down to the task(s) … you break them down into smaller tasks if you want to … but you get on with them … you start them … you continue them and you finish them … and the best thing of all is that you get this wonderful sense of satisfaction while you are doing them … even the merest hint of an internal voice saying 'I don't feel like doing this' only serves to increase your determination to … *do it now and finish it now* … nothing will stop you now … nothing will get in your way … what a tremendous feeling of satisfaction!

Last minute adrenaline blocker
Now you have downloaded this application you will find that you *recognise the faulty thinking of the 'work better under pressure adrenaline junkie'* … that old way causes more *mistakes* without enough focus to notice them or enough time to rectify them … you recognise that this can cause more problems in the long run … for other people even if not for yourself … so from now on *you plan the time needed for a specific task/project … you allow time for review and possible revision of work … you start jobs in plenty of time* … bearing in mind emergencies/glitches/unavoidable delays/… you train yourself simply to *be more disciplined* and *start work on time when you are feeling calm* … you learn to *appreciate that feeling of calm and focus* and *enjoy working in a calm, concentrated and structured way* … you *appreciate the benefits yourself* and *you will be noticing just how much other people appreciate the benefits too.*

This 'application' is for people who claim to like working under the pressure of a deadline but often work ineffectively or create problems for others because they run short of time

Sidetrack blocker
Now you have downloaded this application you will find that you are more and more able to *stay focused on the task in hand* … it becomes second nature to you now to *resist getting sidetracked whatever the temptation* … you hear your internal voice reminding you that 'you want to finish the task in hand

This 'application' is for people who become sidetracked by distractions

223

even more' ... hear those words now 'whatever the temptation, I want to finish this task even more' ... you find you are able to *say 'No' to any unnecessary request ... say 'No' to any pleasurable time waster* ... you *stop all escape routes* ... you *organise your emails* ... you *turn away from distractions* ... you *concentrate on the important task in hand ... completely refusing even to contemplate any other unimportant task* ... you *stay on track* ... you do everything it takes to *stay on track until completion* and then *you have that wonderful feeling of satisfaction* ... a job well done and finished on time!

> Personalise this section with relevant suggestions. Check out beforehand that these suggestions would be in line with what is needed, what is feasible in their specific circumstances

Wisdom Wizard is for any personal reason not accounted for in the other options

And here is an icon that you can click on for fixing a problem that you simply have no conscious idea how to solve ... It's called the Wisdom Wizard, and all you have to do is to click on it ... download it ... and all the wisdom of your unconscious mind will set about fixing it for you ... it can all happen at the unconscious level ... amazingly ... without your conscious mind knowing exactly how it's happening ... it just knows that *something different is happening* ... and, of course, *it is* ... your unconscious is finding appropriate strategies to *'fix' the problem* ... it is re-sorting ... recategorising ... refining strategies so that *from now on you simply find that you are doing things the way you need to ... the way you want to ... on time ... in time* ... and let's face it ... it was about time too! Well done.

> The Wisdom Wizard allows problems to be solved at the unconscious level when there is no conscious solution available

Speaking in Groups, Meetings, Conferences, Classrooms

Variations, Adaptations and Recommendation

You might like to consider first using a script from the *Anxiety, Panic, Phobias* section if the client is having panic attacks at the prospect of their forthcoming presentation or classroom observation. If there has been an unsuccessful, or even disastrous, previous experience, a *Rewind procedure* or *Desensitisation procedure* would be particularly useful. Making use of the script *Confidence anchor* would also be an excellent element to include in your treatment session.

Using a hand levitation or cataleptic hand induction gives an impressive example of the power of the mind and is particularly apt for this type of situation where the client needs to be completely convinced that they have the power and control to carry it off.

The script *Confident presentations* could easily be adapted and used for most kinds of public speaking occasions whether for workplace or social contexts. It would also be useful to use extracts from the script *Calm and confidence* for spoken examinations.

Confident presentations

This script is easily adapted to any kind of public speaking.

You've been telling me how for very many reasons you have decided that now is the time ... really the time to *put all anxieties behind you* and learn how to *speak easily and confidently in any situation* ... *speak easily to any group of people whether they are small groups ... large groups or simply to people in a meeting.*

Important to embed the command of their desired outcome and emphasise this with your voice

Now normally people use notes in some shape or form to act as a prompt for what they need to say and these are exceptionally useful ... but it seems that you have also been making use of some other kinds of notes that are far from useful ... much more like a mental document with stage directions on how to make yourself feel nervous when you gave a talk/ made a presentation ... that you have been carry-ing out to the letter and causing yourself all kinds of hassle/difficulty/anxiety that you can well do without ... so in a few moments' time you can *go on a docu-ment search inside yourself* for these notes so they can be dealt with in the most appropriate way ... so as I count down from 5 to 1 ... you can begin your search to recover this document ... perhaps it is in the filing cabinet of your mind or it might be in the computer of your mind.

Seeds the idea that notes in the form of a prompt sheet are the most useful

Make use of their own language to increase the effect

5 beginning your search ... it seems that a bright light is illuminating everything in *your unconscious* ... and making it easy to see ... 4 everything becoming easily accessible now ... 3 opening the filing cabinet and checking through the folders manually or doing a search for the relevant folder in your PC ... 2 that's it opening the folder ... and 1 searching through the documents ... that's it [Pause] and when you've found it ... please let me know/nod your head ... Good ... now when you quickly scan through it you will find all the old directions there for worries and negative 'what ifs' in your head ... so an interesting

Emphasise the words *'your unconscious'* **to exploit the sound/meaning ambiguity** ... *'you're unconscious'*

Note the presupposition that you will find it 'when you've found it' **i.e. *when* and not *if***

by-product that we discover is that *your mind is a very good learner* … but it was learning the wrong things … so what you need to do right now is to *destroy all those old faulty directions about nerves and worries once and for all* … and *write yourself a new set of notes* which *your quick/smart/sharp mind can learn and follow to the letter* … so that you *give confident presentations in just the way that is right for you* … so now is the time to enjoy taking the paper document and putting it in the shredder … that's right … do it now … switch it on and listen to the sound of every word being shredded and completely destroyed. [Pause] Excellent … what a pleasure! … Or, if you have an original document on your mental computer … please go in and delete it … good … now go immediately to your recycle bin and empty that too … what a relief! … Notice how that feels inside … now you can write new directions where you *plan and organise your talk well in advance* … where you *plan in some practice* at home or with friends for example … and you *experience good confident feelings inside* so that you *speak calmly and confidently* … however few … or however many people are listening and enjoying your presentation.

Reframe

You can make this script more interactive if you prefer, by asking them for feedback on their inner responses

Advance planning is essential for calm and confidence

So now as I count down from 5 to 1 again you will find that … as you *go deeper and deeper* relaxed … *your unconscious* mind not only *becomes more creative* but also simply *absorbs all the positive ideas* you want without your having to do anything at all with your conscious mind except just *allow it all to happen* at the unconscious level … so ready … 5 … notice yourself noticing that wonderful sensation as you go deeper … 4 … notice yourself noticing what creativity feels like inside … 3 … notice how positive thoughts are already being absorbed as you hear the numbers … 2 …taking you deeper and ever more receptive … and all the way down to 1 … that most wonderfully receptive place in you.

Additional deepener with more embedded suggestions for increased receptivity, creativity and ability of the unconscious mind to absorb positive ideas without conscious involvement in the process

From now on you will be using a new set of directions at the unconscious level for speaking in public ... so let's write those right ... now ... ones that will enable you to *get a feeling of enthusiasm* when you begin to think of the presentation/speech you are going to give and a desire to *get down to planning and structuring of the talk straight away* and ... as you do this ... you will discover a positive sense of already being well prepared and in control ... you *carry out all the research you need in good time* and are *feeling very positive* about sharing this with others/your audience/your colleagues. ... Please, mentally commit all these ideas to your internal set of notes/document so that everything will happen automatically in your conscious behaviour. [Pause] ... Good.

> People often postpone preparation because it makes them anxious even to think about the presentation. This lack of preparation causes more anxiety later so it is essential to get this done in good time

Let's continue ... every day *your confidence is growing* in many different areas so that *you think clearly and positively* ... and as you *think clearly and positively* you will notice that you *feel more relaxed and calm inside* ... the idea of *feeling at ease with speaking anywhere ... any time ... with anybody* is something that *is feeling increasingly natural* and is something that *you want to do* ... Every mental 'what if' is focused on positive performance ... what if I enjoy it? ... What if I speak easily and fluently? ... What if I feel really confident? ... And of course all of this leads to the fact that *you are increasingly sleeping well* and *waking refreshed and clear thinking* in the morning ... (please, keep typing/writing this into your internal notes) ... and from now on you will be aware ... at a deep inner level ... of a strong, calm confident feeling in your head ... in your chest ... in your stomach as you go about your everyday life.

> Suggestions for good sleep are important

> Mention the areas in the body where the client experiences anxiety

All of these ideas and feelings have been becoming so much a part of you that on the day of your presentation you will wake refreshed after a good night's sleep with a sense of forward momentum to the day ... on the way to the meeting/the event/the conference you are aware that you have a positive

> A common time for anxiety to build

feeling about the day ahead ... as soon as you enter the hall/room/meeting you will notice a sense of confident excitement ... and you will recognize that this feeling of excitement is going to give you energy and enthusiasm for your talk.

Reframe nervousness as excitement

And as soon as it is your turn to speak your internal automatic switch flicks onto outward focus for the whole duration of your talk ... that's good ... and you will remain completely focused on what you want to say ... you speak with evident ease and confidence that comes from an internal positive belief and conviction deep within you at the unconscious level ... your body reflects this ease as your body is relaxed and natural ... your legs are steady and strong ... your hands are steady and strong.

Outward focus is of paramount importance so they don't focus on their feelings

Common fears are that legs will give way and hands will shake

As you look out at your audience ... you will notice with pleasure that they are looking at you in a friendly way and are interested in what you have to say ... you get a sense of warmth and interest from their eyes ... it makes you feel good each time you look at them ... as you are reminded somehow of the look of friends when they are interested in the conversations that you have with them so easily and naturally ... (they are here because they really want to listen to you).

People often feel that audience eyes are hostile and judgemental and so avoid eye contact

The bracketed phrase is helpful but be sure it applies in the individual case

You think calmly and clearly ... actually enjoying what you have to say ... you speak fluently and with a natural command of your subject whether you are talking to friends, colleagues, your managers or people who report to you ... you are talking with an ease and enthusiasm that is infectious so it may only be later ... as you think back ... that you become aware how your voice was strong and animated.

As your confidence grows you find the size of the group is no longer of any particular relevance, since you naturally adapt your style to the group in front of you ... just as you adapt when you speak to one or to two or to three people ... you enjoy the talk/speech/presentation just as you enjoy having a conversation with your friends. Congratulations ... your unconscious mind is indeed truly powerful.

So before we bring this session to a close I'd like you to notice in your mind's eye that ... standing in front of you now is 'the you from a little while into your future' ... who has already absorbed all of these suggestions so deeply and completely ... that several presentations have now taken place very successfully ... just take a step into the shoes of 'this you' now and feel what it is like to *have that confidence inside* that comes from having experienced such success ... and feeling that inner conviction ... please run through a similar presentation/talk/speech in your mind ... with all this confidence allowing you to *actively enjoy this presentation* in just the way you want it to happen. [Pause] Great ... now look again and notice that 'the you' standing in front of you this time ... is the one who has grown even further in both skill and confidence ... for whom speaking in public/presenting/talking in groups/talking at meetings has become just a routine part of what he/she does on a regular basis ... and I invite you to step into the shoes of 'this you' and ... as you run through every little detail of a presentation/speech again ... notice yourself noticing the ease and the normality of speaking fluently, effortlessly, being fully in the moment ... positively enjoying being completely outwardly focused. [Pause] Hey ... is that applause you can hear?!

Well, I think it's time for you to *bring all of those insights and skills and inner confidence back with you into the present moment of [today's date]* so you can *enjoy them here and now* and *enjoy that confidence growing even stronger every day* ... as the days and the weeks and the months pass by ... it becomes so much second nature to you now to *be confident* ... that you don't even have to consciously

'Future pace' success
Presupposition that suggestions have been absorbed

'actively enjoy' **takes one into a far better state than merely not being afraid**

Embedded commands for confidence

remember to *be confident in everything you do* … it just seems to *happen automatically at the unconscious level* … it's all in your notes and you learned them exceedingly well.

So as I count from 1 to 5 … you will feel as though *you are wakening from a refreshing sleep* … or simply rousing from a wonderful state of relaxation where *you have already made some amazing changes which will improve the quality of your life immeasurably and continue to please and surprise you as each day goes by* … with each ascending number you will come wider awake into the present moment of [today's date] … not that you have really been asleep … just deeply relaxed … more and more aware now of how normal wide awake sensations have returned to your body and fully aware of how positive and alert you are in your mind. [Count from 1 to 5.]

Counting up on the in breath from 1 to 5 mirrors the deepeners used earlier in the script. You can include even more lively, positive suggestions if you wish

Teachers/trainers: being observed in the classroom

This script is aimed at teachers or trainers who have lesson observation as part of a final or continuous assessment. It could also be for inspections by their own organisation or a government department responsible for educational standards, for example OFSTED in the UK. Even experienced teachers can work themselves into a frenzy of anxiety before such inspections.

And here ... it's good to reflect on the fact that your conscious mind works so well in all your preparation and planning ... and now you can allow your unconscious mind to work in its rather different way ... I wonder whether you will *find that you enjoy just absorbing these suggestions* as you *relax and listen* to my voice or whether you will focus your attention on every word as you *take on board each suggestion* that will ensure you not only *teach calmly, competently and confidently* but that you *enjoy your classroom observation/examination as well* ... whichever you do it will be perfect for you ... so ready now.

Double bind of comparable alternatives: either choice of *'relax and listen'* or 'focus your attention' leads you to take on board the suggestions

On the day of any observed lesson you will wake refreshed after a good night's sleep with a sense of forward momentum to the day ... on the way to school/college/the training course, you *become aware that you have a positive feeling about the day ahead* ... as soon as you enter the building you will *notice a sense of belonging here* ... *with an inner calm confidence* ... and while you make any necessary preparations, you will *notice that you have a clear sense of concentration on the task in hand* ... and as soon as it's time for you to go to your lesson ... a calm, outward focus will become even stronger so that *your attention is placed firmly on what you want to say, how you will structure the lesson and how you will respond to the students/ children ... they are your focus of attention and your ability to respond naturally and effectively to them will remain with you throughout the lesson/the day/ training session.*

Note the presupposition of 'a good night's sleep'

Include any specific anxiety-provoking situations elicited in the pre-trance discussion

Outward focus prevents concentration on inner nervous feelings

As soon as you walk into the classroom/training room you feel at home/at ease/completely comfortable … you may *become aware … of a little surge of excitement* … this is the energy and enthusiasm needed in the classroom …. there is an internal ease and confidence deep within you at the unconscious level … your body reflects this ease as *your body is relaxed and natural … your legs are steady and strong … your hands are steady and strong … …* and your mind too reflects this ease as you think calmly and clearly … *you speak with evident ease and confidence* with a strong clear voice … feeling completely in the moment and … with this amazingly clear sense of focus … *you love engaging your students in the topic/on the activity* … in fact this ability to *focus on the task in hand* is so well developed that you are able to *disregard any presence that is irrelevant to the task* … you mentally … and temporarily … put the observer/the examiner/your guest to one side for a while … you can disregard them for the moment as you are completely involved in the task/the lesson … you have prepared so well that you are able to *place your attention on the activity and the response of the students/pupils* … and this confidence allows you to *respond to your students/pupils easily and in a completely natural way* … you are fully in the moment and you are enjoying the lesson … *this is your domain and you are enjoying being here …you just feel completely at home …* you look around you and *notice that the students are interested in the task you have set them/what you are saying*.

Because you have planned for different responses and different eventualities you find it both easy and natural to *expect and deal with the unexpected* … in fact as you have planned for the unexpected … everything in a strange kind of way becomes expected and *you handle things expectedly well* … one of the things you have prepared for, of course, is that a student … for one reason or another that may have nothing whatsoever to do with you … may per-

Anxiety is often manifested in weak legs and shaking hands

The ability to temporarily disregard the presence of an observer is of great importance in this situation. Clearly this should only be temporary since, in any post-lesson discussion, attention to the examiner is crucial

Deliberate confusional suggestions around the expected and unexpected

haps be less co-operative than you would like and yet … because *you are prepared for any eventuality … you refuse to let this faze/disturb/upset you in any way* … you *remain cool, calm and collected and respond resourcefully* … you seem to *understand situations intuitively … see things with an amazing clarity … feel at your most clear headed … feel at ease in yourself* … remembering your training and finding those inner resources to *deal with any situation in the best and most appropriate way* … you are able to *deal with any situation coolly, calmly and in a collected way* … your voice is strong and carries a natural authority … you are able to *think on your feet*, responding with ingenuity, with humour, with authority and *make good decisions throughout the lesson/ training session/the whole day.*

I invite you now to notice that … in front of you is the 'you' who … *having absorbed all the suggestions you have heard today* … has already carried out the observed lesson/training very confidently and competently and knows that not only did you *give a very good lesson* but you … and the students … *enjoyed it as well* … this person is the you, of course, from tomorrow/next week … so how about floating into that person and *be there now in the classroom at the end* of the lesson … notice where exactly in your mind and body you are aware that *you have a positive feeling* that you did your best and everything went very well … look at the observer … and you observe their positive look of approval feel how satisfying that is … now track back through the experience and *enjoy all of those high points* again … the way you *handled everything with ease* … how *your timing was spot on* … how *you were feeling a sense of calm but also a sense of energy and enthusiasm* at the same time … how *your voice was strong and clear and you had an air of authoritative competence about you* … go back even further and notice how you had exceptionally *good recall both for facts and effective strategies* … get a sense of the positive atmosphere in the room and once you get back to

Presupposition that the client will have absorbed the suggestions

'Future pacing' the positive experience of carrying out the lesson with all the positive suggestions in place

Tracking back over an experience is a useful technique since you begin with the successful conclusion of the desired outcome

the beginning ... really *enjoy that confidence and surge of excitement as you walked into the room* ... great.

Now just before we finish ... run through it again from beginning to end ... taking all the time you want ... and enjoy every moment all over again ... this time you *know of course from the very beginning that everything will happen just as you want it to* ... since you *remember that you have already done it all so well before* ... and you will do this now just as quickly as you need for your unconscious mind to *absorb every suggestion* that will ensure that *everything will happen just as you want it to* ... just as I say it will ... once you have finished, just let me know ... tell me or nod your head. [Pause until you get the signal] Excellent, now in a few moments time you can begin to reorient to the room, bringing back every insight and every positive suggestion that will let you *enjoy feeling ... thinking and acting calmly and confidently in everything that you do.*

The more often the scene is visualised, the more likely it is that the behaviour will be carried out in real life

Go to a suitable trance reorientation

Tests and Exams

Calm and confidence for spoken examinations

This script shares the same framework as the one for written exams but uses suggestions that are appropriate for oral exams. It is also suitable for use for interviews or any situation involving performance anxiety – with some simple adaptation.

Now you might have heard that the only way to *experience hypnosis* was through the state of relaxation ... and of course that is one way you can do it ... but you may also be interested to know that you can *go into the hypnotic state through gentle curiosity* ... and I know you can *be curious about many different things* ... and everybody can be curious to know how the state of mind affects the body and how the body affects the state of mind ... and how *some simple changes can be so effective* ... and I wonder if you would be sufficiently curious ... and willing ... to *experience a change in the state of your hand and fingers* right now? [Pause] Good ... so I invite you to rest your finger tips very, very lightly on your knees ... that's right ... just like this ... your fingertips barely touching ... and *focus your attention* on just one of those hands ... really focus ... that's right ... keep your gaze on that hand ... just focusing ... listening ...wondering ... becoming more and more curious whether it will be what you see ... or what you hear ... or what you feel ... that will enable you to *achieve that wonderful trance state* where *your confidence in yourself increases* ... I'd like you to *become very aware of the changes you observe in the hand* ... can you notice how ... as you look at the hand ... you may *find changes beginning to happen?* ... It may seem to you that *the hand is becoming fuzzy and blurred* ... yes, fuzzy and blurred ... or curiously ... it may be that the opposite happens ... *you may notice a very defined outline around the hand* ... becoming more and more defined ... interesting ... I'd like you to ... yes, very interesting ... *notice these things* and allow yourself to *experience them*

Embedded commands begin immediately in a deceptively conversational way using the inflection of the voice

Generalisation 'everybody can be curious'

'the body affects the state of mind' seeds the idea that what they are about to experience will affect their state of mind

Demonstrate how to have the fingertips barely touching the knees

Encourage any response you notice by commenting 'yes that's it' 'that's right' 'interesting' 'Mmm'

236

fully … in whatever way they occur … for it may be that you *first experience the visual changes* … or it may be that first of all … as you turn your attention now to the weight of the hand … (*or is it lightness?*) … there is an experience of that *hand feeling lighter and lighter* … the more you *focus your attention on the sensations in the hand, the more apparent those changes seem to be* … in fact … can you *notice the slight tingling in the finger tips?* … And you can be curious as you notice any little movement … any little lifting urge … becoming aware of that *lifting urge* in perhaps one finger … or is it in more than one finger? … Or is it *the thumb first* that is wanting to lift higher and higher? … Or is it *all the fingers* … as the lightness spreads back into the knuckles? … A light buoyant feeling now beginning in the palm … and is the whole hand now feeling lighter as the urge to *lift higher and higher* is *becoming irresistible* … as if the hand *has a confident mind* of its own … as if it can decide all by itself that it *will* lift higher *and higher* as if it's floating … as indeed it *can* float … *all on its own … higher and higher … all on its own at the unconscious level.* And as you continue to observe the hand floating and lifting all on its own … aware of the experience of the change in perception of your hand … you may also become aware of the positive change in your own inner confidence as you now *begin to notice the feeling of heaviness in your eyelids* … how, as *the hand gets lighter and lighter* … you can *feel that heaviness developing in your eyelids* … heavier and heavier … as the urge for them to *close* becomes more insistent now … that's right … allowing that *wonderful sense of relief to spread over you* as the *eyelids close now* and you *develop that even deeper sense of calm hypnotic relaxation.*

And as you allow this deepening to occur you can consider the power of your unconscious mind in taking control of the movement of the hand and the arm … how amazing it is … this is the power of the trance state that allows your mind and body

'*the* hand' and '*that* hand' **encourages dissociation and a deeper trance state**

There are several phrases in this section which encourage dissociation and depth of the trance state, e.g. *'the thumb' 'all the fingers'* '**the hand** *has a confident mind* **of its own'** '**can decide all by itself'**

The very act of hand levitation has an extraordinarily convincing effect. Being convinced of the power of the unconscious mind is vital in the case of performance anxiety

Links a change in the perception of the hand to a change in perception of more positive confidence

For best effect, synchronise your suggestions for heaviness and closure to the blinking of the eyes

Further reinforcement of the concept of the power of the trance state

to work in harmony to *achieve the level of calm and confidence that is perfect for passing exams.* And as your unconscious mind recognizes now its total readiness for accepting fully and completely the suggestions for calm and confidence before, during and after your exam/exams/test/performance … your arm will begin to feel heavier and heavier too … just like your eyelids. [Pause] That's right … just like that … your arm, sinking down again towards your lap … yes … *you are completely ready to accept.*

Deliberate use of the word 'passing' **exams rather than** '**taking**'

Links the readiness to accept the suggestions with the heaviness of the arm

Comment on, and so ratify, any downward movement

These things will happen in this way through the amazing power of your own mind in the trance state which has already been demonstrated to you. These are the suggestions that will *change your state of mind into a state of positivity … feel yourself accepting them now* … you know you have put in the work and you know you are fully competent … and because you have done this work and because *you are fully aware that you have the required knowledge and facts/vocabulary stored deeply in your memory* … you can also *know that you will access all this information whenever and wherever it is required* … and because *you are very sure of that,* you will find that you *feel calm and confident and at ease about your exam(s)* … you *think clearly, calmly and confidently and you speak easily and fluently before, during and after the exam is successfully completed* … and you *behave calmly and in a cool and composed way all through the lead up … and all the way through, and even after the exam* as you await the results with equanimity … knowing *you have done your very best.*

Powerful suggestion and reminder of the hand levitation

Several direct suggestions are linked together

If this is a foreign language oral exam, the word '**vocabulary**' **will be more appropriate than** 'facts'

So now … with these most positive suggestions deeply embedded in your unconscious mind … I invite you to float into your future now and take a look at yourself and how things are going so well on the day(s) of the exam(s) … notice how …as you *wake from a really good night's sleep* on the morning of your exam, *you are looking and feeling so well*

Presupposition that the suggestions have been accepted

'**Future pace**'

rested and calm ... and then ... there you are ... actually eating breakfast for energy to sustain you ... without a care in the world ... you *continue to feel calm in your mind and at ease in your body all day long* ... before, during and after your exam ... as you travel to the examination you find your mind is drifting onto something pleasant (look, is that a smile on your face?) and look at you as you're arriving ... don't you look calm and confident!

See how you're calmly sitting and waiting patiently for your turn and now ... the moment you walk into the room ... you immediately experience a wonderful feeling of deep inner confidence ... a calm and comfortable feeling in your stomach ... an ease in your breathing ... legs are steady and strong and you have an alert focus in your mind ... and you remember how well you can *focus your attention*, don't you? *As you go in, you look at the examiner and smile ... you have an amazing sense of wanting to put that person at ease ... can* you see that expression of confidence on your face and easy relaxed body language? ... And such clarity of mind! ... You think clearly and well as you look at your examiner in a very friendly and natural way ... staying calm, focused and in control. Any time you want a little extra calm and confidence, you simply glance at your hand *for a split second* ... looking up immediately ... and ... at the unconscious level there is a physical reminder of the wonderful sense of calm and confidence you have been experiencing today ... feel that sense of calm now spreading all the way through you, all the way through your body ... with confident thoughts in your mind ... this is the sense of calm and confidence you will experience any time you glance at your hand for a split second ... your unconscious mind will remind you. That's right ... *glance at your hand and feel calm, steady, comfortable and focused ... look up again immediately ... you feel so good.* Brilliant.

Adapt the following suggestions to build an exam scenario which is appropriate to your client

Picks up the suggestion for focus that was seeded in the induction

Deliberate suggestion of wanting to put the *examiner* at ease. Slightly surprising suggestions are often very effective

Anchors calm and confidence to a split second glance at the hand

Repetition of anchor

There is an inner awareness of calm, confidence and composure which feels so natural in your body ... so good in your mind ... your voice is strong and has good expression and you can hear the enthusiasm shining through ... your thoughts flow easily and the words flow easily ... *you are naturally calm and in control and you are completely outwardly focused. ... The more you were even to try to think of yourself the more you would find yourself being drawn back to focus on the topic ...* you stay on track all the way through ... you feel good, you feel calm and you channel any extra energy into alert focus that helps your concentration and fluent conversation. How well you're doing all of this ... you are obviously enjoying yourself ... I wonder if that surprised you or just felt completely normal and natural ... Congratulations!

The law of reversed effect

What a great result! So, bringing that knowledge of your ability to *behave in exactly the best exam way* ... in a moment or two it will be the time for you to begin to return to the present moment and reorient to the room, bringing with you all that calm, confidence and composure ... *secure in the knowledge that it will stay with you ... inside you ... wherever you are ... whenever you want it ... whatever you want it* for ... it will be there.

What a great result! **Ambiguous comment suggests success in the exam as well as in the guided visualisation**

Go to a suitable trance reorientation and remember to remove all inappropriate sensations of lightness or heaviness induced in the hands, arms and eyelids

Calm and confidence for written examinations

This script shares the same framework as the one for spoken exams but uses suggestions that are appropriate for written exams, including selecting questions, making notes, planning time and staying on track.

Now you might have heard that the only way to *experience hypnosis* was through the state of relaxation … and of course that is one way you can do it … but you may also be interested to know that you can *go into the hypnotic state through gentle curiosity* … and I know you can *be curious about many different things* … and everybody can be curious to know how the state of mind affects the body and how the body affects the state of mind … and how *some simple changes can be so effective* … and I wonder if you would be sufficiently curious … and willing … to *experience a change in the state of your hand and fingers* right now? [Pause] Good … so I invite you to rest your fingertips very, very lightly on your knees … that's right … just like this … your finger tips barely touching … and *focus your attention* on just one of those hands … really focus … that's right … keep your gaze on that hand … just focusing … listening …wondering … becoming more and more curious whether it will be what you see … or what you hear … or what you feel … that will enable you to *achieve that wonderful trance state* where *your confidence in yourself increases* … I'd like you to *become very aware of the changes you observe in the hand* … can you notice how … as you look at the hand … you may *find changes beginning to happen?* … It may seem to you that *the hand is becoming fuzzy and blurred* … yes, fuzzy and blurred … or curiously … it may be that the opposite happens … *you may notice a very defined outline around the hand* … becoming more and more defined … interesting I'd like you to … yes, very interesting … *notice these things* and allow yourself to *experience them fully* … in whatever way they occur … for it may be that you *first experience the visual changes* … or it

Embedded commands begin immediately in a deceptively conversational way using the inflection of the voice

Generalisation 'everybody can be curious'

'the body affects the state of mind' **seeds the idea of what they are about to experience will affect their state of mind**

Demonstrate how to have the fingertips barely touching the knees

Encourage any response you notice by commenting 'yes that's it' 'that's right' 'interesting' 'Mmm'

241

may be that first of all … as you turn your attention now to the weight of the hand … (*or is it lightness?*) … there is an experience of that *hand feeling lighter and lighter* … the more you *focus your attention on the sensations in the hand, the more apparent those changes seem to be* … in fact … can you *notice the slight tingling in the finger tips?* … And you can be curious as you notice any little movement … any little lifting urge … becoming aware of that *lifting urge* in perhaps one finger … or is it in more than one finger? … Or is it *the thumb first* that is wanting to lift higher and higher? … Or is it *all the fingers* … as the lightness spreads back into the knuckles? … A light buoyant feeling now beginning in the palm … and is the whole hand now feeling lighter as the urge to *lift higher and higher* is *becoming irresistible* … as if the hand *has a confident mind* of its own … as if it can decide all by itself that it *will* lift higher *and higher* as if it's floating … as indeed it *can* float … *all on its own … higher and higher … all on its own at the unconscious level.* And as you continue to observe the hand floating and lifting all on its own … aware of the experience of the change in perception of your hand … you may also become aware of the positive change in your own inner confidence as you also now begin to notice the feeling of heaviness in your eyelids … how, as the hand gets lighter and lighter … you can feel that heaviness developing in your eyelids … heavier and heavier … as the urge for them to *close* becomes more insistent now … that's right … allowing that *wonderful sense of relief to spread over you* as the *eyelids close now* and you *develop that even deeper sense of calm hypnotic relaxation.*

And as you allow this deepening to occur you can consider the power of your unconscious mind in taking control of the movement of the hand and the arm … how amazing it is … this is the power of the trance state that allows your mind and body to work in harmony to *achieve the level of calm and*

'*the* hand' and '*that* hand' encourages dissociation and a deeper trance state

There are several phrases in this section which encourage dissociation and depth of the trance state, e.g. '*the thumb*' '*all the fingers*' '*the hand has a confident mind* of its own' 'can decide all by itself'

The very act of hand levitation has an extraordinarily convincing effect. Being convinced of the power of the unconscious mind is vital in the case of examination nerves

Links a change in the perception of the hand to a change in perception of more positive confidence

For best effect, synchronise your suggestions for heaviness and closure to the blinking of the eyes

Further reinforcement of the concept of the power of the trance state *confidence that is perfect for passing exams.* And as your unconscious mind recognizes now its state of readiness for accepting fully and completely the suggestions for calm and confidence before, during and after your exam/exams/test … your arm will begin to feel heavier and heavier too … just like your eyelids. [Pause] That's right … just like that … your arm, sinking down again towards your lap … yes … *you are completely ready to accept.*

Deliberate use of the word 'passing' **exams rather than** 'taking'

Links the readiness to accept the suggestions with the heaviness of the arm

Comment on, and so ratify, any downward movement

These things will happen in this way through the amazing power of your own mind in the trance state which has already been demonstrated to you. These are the suggestions that will *change your state of mind into a state of positivity … feel yourself accepting them now … feel yourself accepting them now* … you know you have put in the work and you know you are fully competent … and because you have done this work and because *you are fully aware that you have the required knowledge and facts stored deeply in your memory* … you can also *know that you will access all this information whenever and wherever it is required* … and because *you are very sure of that,* you will find that you *feel calm and confident about your exam(s)* … you *think clearly, calmly and confidently before, during and after the exam is successfully completed* … and you *behave calmly and in a cool and composed way all through the lead up … and all the way through, and even after the exam* as you await the results with equanimity … knowing *you have done your very best.*

Powerful suggestion and reminder of the hand levitation

Several direct suggestions are linked together

So now … with these positive suggestions deeply embedded in your unconscious mind … I invite you to float into your future now and take a look at yourself and see how things are going so well on the day(s) of the exam(s) … notice how …as you *wake from a really good night's sleep* on the morning of your exam, *you are looking and feeling so well rested and calm* … and then … there you are … actually

Presupposition that the suggestions have been accepted

Future pace

eating breakfast for energy to sustain you ... without a care in the world ... you *continue to feel calm in your mind and at ease in your body all day long* ... before, during and after your exam. ... As you travel to the examination you find your mind is drifting onto something pleasant (look, is that a smile on your face?) and look at you as you're arriving ... don't you look calm and confident!

Adapt the following suggestions to build an exam scenario which is appropriate to your client

Now you're walking in and calmly finding your place ... arranging your things ... now, sitting and waiting steadily and patiently for the signal to begin and ... the moment you turn over the paper/open the booklet ... you immediately experience a slight surge of alert yet calm focus ... and you remember how well you can *focus your attention*, don't you? *As you pick up your pen/pencil ... this focus develops even more* so that you are fully focused as you *read each question through thoroughly*. ... Notice how you are underlining key parts of the question and selecting the best questions to answer ... can you see that expression of concentration on your face? ... And such clarity of mind! ... You think clearly and well as you make notes of key words and phrases relevant to your answer ... look, now you're planning the time required for each answer ... you stick to this time, leaving yourself plenty of time for more challenging questions. Some questions may be more appealing than others ... however you simply *get on with answering the chosen questions unemotionally* ... staying calm, focused and in control. Any time you want any extra calm, you simply glance at your hand *for a split second* ... looking up immediately ... and at the unconscious level there is a physical reminder of the wonderful sense of calm and alert focus you have been experiencing today ... feel that sense of calm now spreading all the way through you, all the way through your body and a crystal clear focus in your mind, this is what you will experience any time you glance at your hand for a split second ... your unconscious mind will remind you. That's right ...

Anchors turning the page to calm and focus

Picks up the suggestion of excellent focus of attention that was seeded in the induction

Key exam strategies

Anchors calm and alert focus to glancing at the hand for a split second

244

glance at your hand and feel calm and steady, alert and focused. Brilliant.

Sometimes you even seem to hear your inner voice reminding you that *you are calm and in control*. You stay on track all the way through … you stick to time … you feel good, you feel calm and you channel any extra energy into alert focus that helps your concentration. How well you're doing all of this … notice how you're nearing the end and you're looking so pleased that you have saved plenty of time to check through your work with calm and care. … Congratulations!

What a great result! So, bringing that knowledge of your ability to behave in exactly the best exam way … in a moment or two it will be the time for you to begin to return to the present moment and reorient to the room, bringing with you all that calm, confidence and composure … and crystal clear focus too … secure in the knowledge that it will stay with you … inside you … wherever you are … whenever you want it … whatever you want it for … it will be there.

'What a great result!'
Ambiguous comment suggests success in the exam as well as in the guided visualisation

Go to a suitable trance reorientation and remember to remove all inappropriate sensations of lightness or heaviness induced in the hands, arms and eyelids

Sport and Performance

Variations, Adaptations and Recommendations

The scripts in this section could be used with other types of performing artists with fairly minimal adaptation. Mental, physical and emotional preparation and constructive evaluation is vital for all, and, unfortunately, rejection and disappointment will be experienced by most at some time in their career. Other scripts which, again with some adaptation, will be found useful are *Confidence anchor*, *Be resilient in the workplace*, *Confident presentations*, and several in the *Anxiety, Panic, Phobias* section (but please note the comment below about the state of calm not always being desirable for athletes and performers).

It is essential to check out individual 'needs and wants' with sportsmen and women and performing artists in general since minimal differences can be critical. Don't assume that their preferred state will be one of calm. There are certainly times when this will be appropriate but there are also many occasions where, particularly in the case of physical performers, they prefer to feel psyched up, on the edge, taut and ready to go.

With most of the scripts in this section a simple light induction would be the most suitable; the client doesn't need to be in a deep trance state and can get a better result with a more alert focused state akin to that of being absorbed in thought.

Selection of coaching questions to be used with the script 'Evaluate and improve performance'

In the dressing room:

- How is your mood?
- What are you saying to yourself?
- How prepared do you feel?
- How fit are you?
- How is your mental attitude?
- How are your emotions?
- How are your emotions affecting you?

- How is your breathing?
- How is your focus and concentration?
- Does it need to be narrowed or expanded at this point?
- Is there anything you need to change at this point to improve things?

On the track/court/field/course/stage:

- How is your mood now?
- What are you saying to yourself?
- How prepared do you feel?
- How fit are you?
- How is your mental attitude?
- How are your emotions?
- How are your emotions affecting you?
- How is your energy?
- How is your focus and concentration?
- Does it need to be narrowed or expanded at this point?
- Is there anything you need to change at this point to improve things?
- What is working well at a technical level?
- What needs to be changed or adjusted?
- Feel the sensation of that stroke/movement/action … what's working/not working?
- What do you need to discuss with your coach/trainer?

After the match/game/performance, having a discussion with your trainer:

- What do you think your trainer/coach would be saying?
- What are you learning about your mood/technique/fitness/concentration?
- What do you have to do to improve your performance?
- What else?

Evaluate and improve performance

In your pre-trance discussion it would be useful to identify two or three main areas for evaluation and improvement so that the client has a defined area of focus. Select questions from the *coaching questions* on pages 250–1 that are appropriate to each stage of the match (pre- and post-match, as well as their performance in the match itself). This script can be used to diagnose problems and be followed up, as required, with other relevant scripts in this section.

I'd like you to cast your mind back to an occasion when you have been able to be particularly objective and to identify problem areas and offer constructive criticism. This may be an occasion related to sport or it may be something completely unrelated but the important thing is that you are making full use of your ability to *be completely objective in your judgement* ... and let me know when you've found that time. [Pause] Good ... let yourself *be there now in your mind and explore how that feels* ... how *your thoughts seem to be crystal clear* ... how *you seem to be able to identify critical details in problem areas* and how *you can find useful solutions*. So let's call this your 'constructive critical ability' and every time you want to make use of this frame of mind you can remind yourself of this ability and call this state to mind.	**Ask your client to identify such an occasion during your pre-trance discussion** **Anchoring the state to use later**
So now I'd like to invite you to bring all this 'constructive critical ability' to bear as you prepare to watch a mental film of your last performance ... see that mental DVD player in your mind's eye ... pick up the DVD and insert it in the player ... feel that remote control in your hand and ... in a moment ... you'll begin to watch ... and as you do I'm going to ask you some questions about your mental attitude on that occasion, your mood and your technical performance ... use your remote control to pause the film as necessary. So, let's start the film in the <u>dressing room</u> ... we'll only move on to the match/performance itself after you've taken everything there is to learn from the <u>dressing room</u> situation ...	**Watching the performance from a dissociated perspective affords a more objective point of view** **Visual and kinaesthetic** **It's useful to find out about their mood before they even begin their performance. Ask the client the best place to begin the film, at home, in the dressing room etc.**

I'm going to ask you a question and give you all the time you need to watch the film … when you have found the answer you can speak easily and clearly while remaining in this highly focused light trance state … and I will make a note of your answer for your future use. I want you to know that you have a zoom lens on your control … so do please zoom in and slow down the film whenever you want to examine it in greater detail … you can rewind and fast forward the film just as often as you need to … so tell me when you can see yourself on screen there in the dressing room. [Pause for as long as needed between questions.]

Select appropriate questions from the list on pages 250–1 and keep a note of their answers

Excellent … and now we'll move onto the match itself … once again using all of your 'constructive critical ability' and remembering that you have your zoom lens whenever you need it … I'm going to ask you some more questions.

Select appropriate questions for the match/performance itself

(*If the client were to get stuck at any point*, you can ask them to put down the remote control and step in and out of the film to get different perspectives, or ask them to put on the trainer's hat for yet a different opinion)

Excellent … now shall we move onto after the event is over and imagine that you are sitting having a discussion with your trainer as you run through that DVD again together … what do you think they have to say? [Pause] Excellent.

Select questions as appropriate

You have done some great evaluation here so I think now is the time for you to *relax a little more deeply* and really enjoy a few more minutes before you drift up into a fully alert state once again … and allow all of this learning here today to fully develop unconsciously … which will naturally show itself later at the conscious level in so many different ways …

Add in a deepener here if you think it would be advantageous to have some deeper relaxation

So relaxing pleasantly here … I invite you to visualise yourself doing your self-hypnosis over the next few days/weeks to improve your mood/control

Assumes you have taught, or will teach, self-hypnosis

your temper/do more fitness training/practise that technique ... and let me know when you've gone through that in some detail. [Pause] Very well done.

Now, I'd like you to visualise yourself going through your next <u>match</u> and with everything happening just as you need it to do ... just as you want it to do ... excellent ... now see yourself doing your post performance routine with your critical yet very constructive hat on ... now feel that sense of real inner satisfaction as you realise that your efforts and hard work are paying off ... well done ... congratulations. So time to switch off the DVD player and ... in a few moments' time ... you can begin that process of reorienting to your surroundings.

Final visualisation of the successful performance

Go to a suitable trance reorientation

Variations, Adaptations and Recommendations

This script can be adapted for use with performing artists of any kind – musicians, singers, actors and dancing – as well as men and women in any sports arena.

Improve your focus and concentration

As you sit there with your hands loosely resting on your lap with your thumbs almost touching ... I'd like you to focus your attention right in the middle of those two hands ... focus your attention on the thumbs ... and ... at the same time ... without moving your eyes at all ... allow yourself to notice all the fingers ... notice the outline of your hands in your peripheral vision ... without moving your eyes at all ... let yourself take in any information that enters your field of vision ... just be aware of how much you can see without moving your eyes at all ... noticing now perhaps that *your vision is becoming rather fuzzy and blurred* ... not moving your eyes at all ... and now begin to concentrate your attention once again just on the thumbs ... keeping your eyes perfectly still ... narrow your attention so you are completely focused on the thumbs ... so you can blot out anything from your line of vision except the thumbs ... that's it ... now noticing that *your eyelids are feeling as if they want to blink* ... wanting to blink ... yes ... *blinking their way closed* ...that's it ... and as soon as your eyes close ... *you will know that you are ready to enter that internal state of concentration* ... where your conscious and your unconscious minds can work together in harmony ... and *increase your ability to narrow or expand your focus at will* ... instantly and effortlessly ... *narrow your focus to the exclusion of everything else or expand your focus to absorb all the information available* ... instantly and effortlessly ... at will ... that's right.

And now allow your mind to *drift back into a time when you were completely focused on the task in hand* ... physically, mentally, emotionally focused on what needed to be done in that moment ... let yourself use all of your senses now to see ... hear ... feel ... think ... behave ... and to react with perfect focus in the way which is right for you ... *be there right now* ... that's right ... everything flowing ... your mind is

This induction makes use of a natural ability to focus and defocus visually and is an appropriate lead into the main body of the script

Visual

Kinaesthetic

Synchronise your comments with their blinking and it will intensify the response

The embedded commands both restate the goal and also give post-hypnotic suggestions for narrowing and expanding focus at will

Anchors positive feelings of focus previously experienced

VAK

fully focused … everything is working perfectly … your body is responding absolutely perfectly … your unconscious and your conscious mind in complete harmony … focused on the task … focused on the moment … to the exclusion of everything else … that's it … and as you *fully enjoy that experience* … say the word FOCUS to yourself … say it mentally or out loud … just as you prefer … you can talk and remain in the state of hypnosis … listen to the word as you say it and discover that you *get that sense of perfect focus* … feel the sensation fully as you say and hear that word … you are completely focused on the task in hand … completely focused on the moment … that's right … this word FOCUS is now so closely associated with this feeling of complete concentration that *whenever you say it … whenever you hear it … your mind and your body will become totally and completely focused … concentrated on the task of the moment.*

You can add in their own descriptions of perfect focus

Install auditory anchor

Now let that concentration relax for a while and allow your mind to drift for a moment or two … just relax comfortably and enjoy the moment … feelings of pleasant calm and relaxation … that's it … enjoy the moment. [Pause] Wonderful … now say the word FOCUS and notice how that state of focus and concentration instantly returns … you see clearly … you think clearly … you get that feeling of your mind and body being in complete harmony and every cell of your being in total alert focus and concentration … that's it and from now on *whenever you say this word … say it aloud or merely say it in your head … this amazing state of alert focus will reappear automatically.*

Allow sufficient time for them to drift off somewhere in their mind

Fire auditory anchor

Post-hypnotic suggestion

You could repeat this section as reinforcement if desired

Sometimes a state of total focus and narrow concentration is exactly what you need and what you want … but it may be that sometimes you need … equally quickly … to expand your peripheral vision and expand your focus ... then all you need to do is to *say the word EXPAND to yourself and automatically your focus is expanded to the exact level you require* ... so I invite you to do this now ... to experiment for a moment or two ... imagine yourself on the court and when the situation requires it ... say the word FOCUS and see, feel, hear your focus narrowing to the exact level you require ... who knows, maybe you even get a smell ... a taste of that focus ... that's it ... and now ... at the exact moment you require it ... say the word EXPAND to yourself and *let all your senses pick up exactly what they need from a wider field of vision* ... a wider sense of feeling ... a wider appreciation of sound to the exact level required ... excellent ... well done.

And every day you can *strengthen and quicken this response by spending just five minutes of your time going over again in your mind this simple exercise* we have just carried out ... and each time you reorient to the room after your practice ... your vision and all your senses will return to optimum functioning ... just as they will do when you reorient to the room in a few minutes' time ... you will see clearly and perfectly ... and you will always be able to narrow and expand your focus according to the circumstances and exact needs of the moment.

Go to a suitable energising trance reorientation

Include specific suggestions if your client has identified very particular times or triggers where such narrow or expanded focus is required. Otherwise leave it to them to mentally fill in the details

Olfactory

Get the client's agreement, both before and after the trance, to carry out this practice

Deal with negativity and stay motivated

For defeat, disappointment, rejection, anger or any negative emotion or lack of energy.

Use the *Ratio breathing* script in the *Inductions* section because the technique is made use of during the script. If you choose not to do so, you will need to adapt that section of the script.

It seems that negative thoughts have been playing on your mind and getting in the way of your perform-ance ... and as you continue your breathing in and breathing out ... in that same pattern as before ... I'd like you to let yourself become aware of any thought that comes to mind ... be, what is called, 'mindful' of that thought and notice that ... if it's unhelpful in any way ... you can simply use your breathing to let that thought go ... and what's even better ... as you breathe it out ... you can choose the best place for it to go.

Typical negative thoughts may focus around disappointment, defeat, anger or frustration at oneself, lack of self-belief

There will be some thoughts that are *unrelated/ irrelevant* and you can just *let those thoughts disperse into the atmosphere* but others can be breathed into a place of transformation ... there's an energising space and a calming space ... there's a forgiving space ... there's a learning space and maybe *some other spaces too that you will find along the way* ... so as you allow those thoughts to come into your head ... just notice them and *direct them into the most appropriate place for you* ... remember that thoughts of anger and frustration have a lot of negative energy that can be very destructive to your game/sport/shot so why not send them to the space that harnesses and trans-forms that energy into something positive which will work *for* you rather than *against* you? So notice any such angry thoughts now and breathe them into the space for transforming and making use of that energy ... notice the fire in the thought and in the feeling ... any colour ... any sensation ... any characteristic ... as you let it flow right out of you

Personalise the script with allusions to any specific types of thought relevant to the client

Many serious sports people are accustomed to the idea of harnessing negative energy so this should fit into their model of the world

… so it can leave you more comfortable, calm and relaxed … with a sense of satisfaction that all of that energy can be put to positive use … and now use all your senses to *transform that energy into something positive* … see it … feel it … (maybe you can hear as well as feel the vibration?) … And attach some positive thoughts to this new energy … 'I will use all of this energy in a very positive way … it will give me power … I have all the power I need … each time anything angers or frustrates me I will transform it into positive power that I can feel within … I have all the energy I need.' Excellent!

And you also told me that you frequently had a tendency to beat yourself up for mistakes that you made … torturing yourself … hanging onto those mistakes long after you should have let them go … either during or after the match/game etc. is over … so right now let any of those thoughts and feelings about mistakes past, present or future be breathed into the forgiveness space … and in this space attach a thought to them … 'I will forgive myself for this mistake/poor performance … I will forgive myself for this error/poor performance because I can *learn from it and do something positive with it*' … take a moment now and once you have forgiven yourself … breathe the mistakes into the learning zone … and stand back and notice in a detached way exactly what you can learn from each of them. … What is there to learn on a very practical level … in a very detailed and objective way? [Pause] And what is there that you can learn at the emotional level … how much of that mistake, for example, was caused by letting yourself become immersed in the emotion? [Pause] What else is there to learn? [Pause] That's good … very good.

Allow them to answer you out loud or mentally and privately as they prefer

Now let your whole self drift into the calming zone and once again do your ratio breathing and notice how it calms you even quicker than before … In 2, 3 … Out 2, 3, 4, 5, 6 … In 2, 3 … Out 2, 3, 4, 5, 6 … and *each time you breathe out through your nose,*

Ratio breathing

255

you can breathe out any tension in your body ... you can even look inside and notice the colour of that tension and ... as we count ... just breathe out that colour ... Out 2, 3, 4, 5, 6 ... *breathe away any tension in your mind ... that's right ....* breathing In 2, 3 ... Out 2, 3, 4, 5, 6 ... In 2, 3 ... Out 2, 3, 4, 5, 6 ... and *each time you do this ... your level of inner calm and comfort increases ...* you *become more and more calm ... you become more and more in control of your relaxation ... and your unconscious mind becomes more and more attentive and receptive to the positive suggestions that are so right for you.*

So just let that calming breathing continue while your unconscious mind absorbs these affirmations deep into your innermost self ... repeat them silently to yourself now ... 'I am calm ... I am positive ... I think rationally, clearly and objectively ... I believe in myself ... I am very able to achieve my goals ... I will stay optimistic and I will focus exclusively on the exact task in hand ... I believe in myself ... I have all the energy and stamina I need and I have all the determination I need ... I will transform any anger or frustration into positive energy ... I will remain totally focused on the exact task of the moment ... I believe in myself.'

Include specific suggestions that your client has identified as important during your discussion. Leave plenty of pauses for them to repeat the affirmations to themselves

And now isn't it good to know that you can bring these thoughts back when you want them ... when you need them ... by simply using the power of your unconscious mind ... all you have to do is simply to practise this breathing technique for a few minutes every day as agreed ... and nobody knows better than you do the importance and the value of regular practice ... and each time you do it ... you will become more and more proficient so that very soon indeed you will find that this has become an invaluable tool ... an instant trigger for calm ... that you can use on court/on the course/on the track etc ... all you will need to do then is to use your breathing ... you will become so proficient that you

Sportsmen and women understand the value of practice and will normally diligently carry out the instruction for daily practice

will only need to *take a breath (and count to three ... that's all you need ... and breathe out from one to six) ...* that's all you need ... and *automatically all unwanted, unhelpful thoughts will be breathed into the appropriate zone and transformed ... quite automatically ...* you will have all the calm/focus/ you need ... you will have all the energy you need ... you will have each of these in exactly the right proportion for the time and the occasion ... that's right ... your thoughts will be powerful and positive ... that's perfect.

If the nature of the sport allows the ratio breathing, use the command of 'in to 3 etc., otherwise merely refer to a simple in breath

It is important to stress 'exactly the right proportion for the time and the occasion' **since very different states may be appropriate at different stages of the match etc**

Take a moment now to see yourself on the court/ the course/the pitch/the track etc. and observe that when something occurs that *might once* have trig- gered that unwanted thought/feeling/response ... now you merely take a breath (breathe in to three and out to six) and you automatically transform your thoughts and feelings into those that are empower- ing which create exactly the state you need ... that's it ... feel that unwanted thought float away and enjoy that sense of calm/energy/positivity/focus etc.

The implication of 'might once' **is that this will no longer occur**

If the nature of the sport allows the ratio breathing, use the command of 'in to 3 etc., otherwise merely instruct them to take a single breath

Use resources specifically suggested by the client. They understand their needs

From now on you will be able to pick up your mood whenever you need to ... whether this is before, dur- ing or after the game/match/event. If it is afterwards, you will allow yourself an appropriate time to reflect and recover ... then you will pick up your mood, move forward, take each experience as a valuable piece of learning, store it away where it is readily available to you when you need it ... and you will be eager to move forward ... you will have a great sense of eager anticipation. So in a few moments it will be time for you to reorient to the surroundings ... feeling refreshed and reinvigorated.

It is necessary to take some time to work through natural disappointment, but a sportsperson needs the ability not to prolong this and to pick up their motivation once again

Go to an energising trance reorientation

Self-belief

Use a light, focusing induction technique.

Remember to read this through before use so as to have the appropriate discussion beforehand.

Everyone has different abilities and positive beliefs about themselves both in the context of sport and also in our wider lives ... and sometimes we have doubts and fears too ... that's normal but the very important thing is to *make use of all your powerful beliefs and abilities when you practise and when you play a match* ... this is the time for you to *believe in yourself* ... so I'd like you to become aware in your mind's eye of a special sports bag ... this is not your normal sports bag ... this is one where you are going to store any doubts, fears or negative beliefs about yourself or your game ... see it there on the bench ... notice what colour it is ... check it has a strong zip ... check it's waterproof ... you have that image in front of you? Now touch it and get the feel of it ... the material ... the zip ... perhaps it has a smell? That's it ... just open it up and have it there beside you on the bench.

Use whichever terminology is appropriate to the client's sport of course

Encourage use of all the senses

Now let yourself become aware of any negative or unhelpful thought, doubt or opinion about yourself in any sphere whatsoever and as it comes to mind ... place it in that sports bag ... I'm not asking you to deny it (although you might like to assess it and *do that another time*) ... for the moment ... simply place it in the bag and keep going until there are none left inside you ... they are all in the bag ... let me know when they're all there ... good ... this is quite simply not the time or the place for them ... now zip up that bag and walk over to the locker ... stow it away ... lock the door and put the key somewhere for safe keeping ... let me know when you've done that ... great! This is quite definitely not the time or the place for any of them ... you can come back and open up the bag when you want to and *deal with any of those contents in the most appropriate way* but when you train/practise/play/perform ... you always stow them away in this bag and put them in the locker so they are unable to get out. Let me know when you understand and agree with that absolutely. Great stuff!

Now I would like you to consider your very positive qualities and abilities ... you can go through them in your mind or you can say them out loud if you like ... whichever way is good for you ... take all the time you need and let me know when you've done that if you are doing it silently and mentally. [Pause] Excellent. Now I would like you to see in your mind's eye your typical sporting gear and place those positive thoughts and abilities within ... in your shoes ... in your tee shirt ... in your shorts ... your track suit ... speak the thought in your mind as you do it ... you may want to see yourself and feel yourself sewing them inside the garment ... Inhale the positivity associated with the smell of the clothes ... excellent.

From now on whenever you train or play, always leave yourself time to sit down quietly, calmly and focus your mind ... and ... as you *carry out this powerful mental exercise* ... you will find that *the moment you walk out on court, you feel positive, upbeat, and you believe absolutely in yourself ... you know you have the power ... you know you have the energy ... you know you have the attitude and you know you have the ability to focus and concentrate on the* moment ... concentrate on the particular task in hand at every given moment throughout the game/match/training. Each time you do this, you will strengthen the effect ... you will strengthen your mental attitude and you will strengthen your game.

Go to a suitable trance reorientation

Allude to qualities elicited in the pre-induction talk such as determination, focus and strength

Link a positive anchor to their clothes. Check they understand this refers to *all* sports clothes they wear

Encourage use of all the senses

Get their agreement to do this beforehand

Leave the pain beside the court

Dissociation

This script was originally written for a tennis player, hence the title; nevertheless it can be used for any sports activity. It deals with a state of *temporary dissociation from pain* during a match. It is essential, prior to use of the script, to establish that your client is playing in compliance with medical advice. An adapted form of this script is also to be found in *Leave the pain beside you* in the *Coping with Pain* section.

Now you are feeling more comfortably relaxed ... so comfortable and relaxed that there are times when you're hardly aware of your body at all ... totally absorbed in listening to the sound of my voice taking you into an even more creative and receptive state of mind ... you can begin to address the purpose of your visit ... to find a way for you to *play your match/ go into the ring/run your race to the very best of your ability* ... *with the very smallest amount of aware- ness of any uncomfortable sensation in your elbow/ ankle/knee that would be necessary for you to stay safe* ... ... *you will of course have your normal excel- lent awareness in every other respect* ... and isn't it reassuring to know that in the state of hypnosis your mind and body can work amazingly well in harmony to *allow all this to occur* ... just as you want it to ... just as you need it to ... and you know ... better than anyone ... how you have already used your mind to *direct attention away from your body* when you've needed to ... when a part of you, for example was hurting or aching and just needed a rest ... and yet you simply used your mind to *direct attention away from your body* ... you may have done this consciously or unconsciously ... or even both ... but somehow you were able to *convince your body that it had enough energy* and it had enough power to *continue right through to the end of the match* ... and so you did. Of course, *sportsmen and women are particularly good at this* ... but even people with- out your training and commitment are able to *carry*

Restates the goal, which concentrates the mind, but also provides the opportunity to embed appropriate commands

For their safety they need to retain a certain amount of awareness

Emphasise *'your normal excellent awareness in every other respect'*

Reminds them of their own ability and also embeds the necessary command *out quite amazing things on occasion* … think of those examples we've all read about where a person is able to *find a kind of superhuman strength* to lift a vehicle and release someone trapped beneath it … or someone badly injured has managed to carry a companion to safety and only notice their own injuries after the event is over … and because of the power of the mind … were able to *do this safely* so this is an ability *we all have inside us when we really need it* … and you have told me that you really need to go out on court … both in training and for the match itself … and *play with all your skill and flair and energy* … (and you have also reassured me that medical opinion says it is safe for you to do this as long as you have adequate rest and treatment prior to and after the tournament).

Now that pain you have been experiencing in your arm/leg/foot/thigh was there for a very good reason … its purpose was to alert you to the fact that your arm/leg/foot/thigh needs rest/medical attention/treatment … and you are very aware of that … you have already taken advice and have already taken steps to *ensure that you get that treatment* and … as you have been told that it is safe for you to play and ignore the pain/discomfort … this is what you will do in a rather unusual way … I'd like you to become aware of that pain as having a kind of personality in its own right … and you could have a bit of a chat with it … just silently in your mind now … and you can of course use your own words to *do it* … just explain that you fully respect its protective purpose for you and that you are definitely going to have the appropriate treatment … and so … because its purpose has been fulfilled/its advice has been heeded … ask it to *take a break while you are playing* and only *reappear after the match/game/ event* to double-check that you really *do get the necessary treatment* … fine … just do that now … mentally and silently and let me know when you've done it. [Pause] Good. Thank you.

Reminds them of amazing feats that human beings can achieve through the power of the mind and also embeds commands

A generalisation

Draws attention to safety procedures. Adapt this to the circumstances of your client

Talk to the part responsible for the pain and reframe. Acknowledge and respect its protective role

Now here's the plan ... the moment you walk out onto the court/the field/the pitch the pain, the sensation can float out of your body and sit there on the sideline watching you ... its role is to *experience any possible discomfort outside your body* so that *nothing bothers you ... nothing disturbs your concentration* ... that part over there can experience any necessary sensations ... right over there ... completely away from you ... and allow you to play your match comfortably ... you will know it's there but it *doesn't bother you at all* ... you can remain entirely comfortable throughout ... that part over there on the sidelines has two responsibilities in protecting you ... one is to experience any sensations outside of your body so that *you yourself needn't be aware of it at all* ... and the second responsibility is to be aware that ... at any time when you truly need to be alerted to danger to yourself ... its job would be to step back into your body and give you a warning so you can *safeguard yourself* ... so just take another moment or two just silently within yourself ... to check that 'your pain part' is agreeable to this plan and then we will move to the final part of the session. [Pause]

'the sensation can float out of your body' **encourages dissociation**

'that part over there on the sidelines' **encourages further dissociation**

A safety precaution

Excellent. All that remains for now ... and also every day until the match ... is some mental practice to ensure that everything happens just as you want it to ... and as a sportsman/sportswoman, *you of all people, will be absolutely aware of the importance of continuing practice in determining success* ... and the mental exercise is for you to is to *imagine that you are watching a training film of you* ... can you see it? Good ... look at you walking out onto the court/the field/the pitch and ... as you do ... you look up and you notice how *there is a part of you that is floating up and out of you* ... *right over there to sit down and make itself very comfortable on the sidelines* ... what does that part look like I wonder as it settles down to watch you *play magnificently* while it does whatever it needs to do to *keep you safe* ... *keep you comfortable and strong* ... *keep you*

Repetition of the imagery is essential and sports people above all others will be aware of the importance of this

Observation of the dissociation

'what does that part look like?' **encourages further dissociation**

flexible and at ease all the way through the match … look at you … nothing bothers you … nothing disturbs your concentration … you are completely focused … you are magnificent!

And once its job is done … so amazingly well … that part of you that has been on guard … experiencing any necessary sensations for you on the outside … so as to keep you as comfortable as can be … will automatically float back into your body … so that all parts of you are fully integrated … your mind and body in harmony … now feeling positive and pleased with a very successful outcome … and also comfortably reassured that you have a part of you … that can keep you safe … both by letting appropriate sensations indicate that something needs attention if and when necessary … and also … at your own request … by protecting you from unwanted sensa-tion when it is safe for it to do so … a very special ability indeed.

Reintegration of parts

Go to an energising trance reorientation

Miscellaneous

Cope with having dyslexia

Having dyslexia often has a negative effect on self-esteem since experience has taught those with the condition to compare themselves unfavourably with others. This is often compounded over time by attitudes of peers, teachers and employers and sometimes even family members. It often makes life tiring and more of a struggle in general as they have problems not only with reading and spelling but with general organisation and time management too. The script focuses on changing harmful self-denigrating beliefs, increasing their belief in their ability to learn and increasing self-confidence. It is not about teaching them to spell.

You've told me that you've been finding it difficult and tiring to cope with having dyslexia so this may be just the right time to take a break and relax a little … so why not take the opportunity right now to let your mind do nothing more than *drift off* to a soothing, calming place where you can notice that your gentle breathing can deepen your relaxation *and increase your comfort*.

And with each breath you take, with each word you hear … you can allow that feeling of physical comfort to deepen … and … you can use your breathing to relax your whole body … with each out breath … let all your muscles relax … starting in your scalp … your forehead … your head … and as you do … let go of anxiety and limiting self-doubt associated with those old tense feelings … that's it … let all your muscles relax … now let all the tension release from the back of your neck and shoulders with the out breath … all the way down your arms and hands and out through the tips of your fingers … and as you do … let go of any old uncomfortable thoughts and feelings associated with that tension in your neck and your shoulders that has been inhibiting you from expressing yourself in the way that you want … that's it … let all your muscles relax … now let all the tension release

This progressive relaxation deepener links the relaxing of muscles to release of specific negative thoughts associated with tension in different parts of the body. You can include any references here to personal information elicited in your pre-trance discussion. Using the client's own language will make the script more effective

all the way down your spine … and as you do … let go of any old uncomfortable thoughts and feelings associated with that tension that has been weighing you down … that's it … let all your muscles relax … now let all the tension release from the muscles in your chest and down through the trunk of your body … and as you do … let go of any old uncomfortable thoughts and feelings associated with those feelings of tightness and restraint that has been restricting you … that's it … let all your muscles relax … now let all that unwanted tiring, tension release all the way down through your legs … down through your knees … down through your ankles and into your feet and out through the very tips of your toes … and as you do … let go of any old uncomfortable thoughts and feelings associated with that tension that has been stopping you from moving forward … that's it … let all your muscles relax … what a relief … and find yourself becoming aware of how much more relaxed and free you feel.

It's wonderful that you've been letting go of all the tiring/exhausting tension that you'd been holding inside for so long … and that letting go will continue with each out breath … and now … you can *take a deep in breath* and begin to *balance your body and mind with ease and a bit of positivity* … you can feel it balancing your body and mind … and listen to your thoughts as you begin to remember some of the things that you enjoy … some of the things that you are good at … maybe listening to music that you love or singing or dancing or playing sport … perhaps remembering a time when you designed or constructed something and were really proud of what you'd done? Or had a brilliant original idea? Or maybe you helped a friend … or were particularly thoughtful and loving to friends, a partner or family … maybe you are loyal, kind and get on with people … you probably already know that some of the most successful people, some of the *real entrepreneurs* are the ones that were not particularly academic … or possibly didn't even enjoy school at all … but they

Mention anything relevant that you have elicited in your pre-trance discussion

You could mention any current well-known entrepreneur who would be an appealing role model to your client

265

have amazing ideas … they're enthusiastic … good at getting on with people and *all of these things are very valuable indeed … just as **you** are very valuable indeed* … so just *continue letting your in breath remind you of strengths and positive resources that you do have* … and let it fill your lungs and let it spread all around your body and mind now … and this can continue as you *continue to relax deeper and deeper as you listen.*

And in this comfortable slightly dreamy state I want to talk to you about your mind, *which actually is so incredibly creative and full of potential* … we all have our conscious mind that we use actively to think and work things out … and we all have our unconscious mind that acts as a storehouse of information and knowledge … stores memories, feelings, habits and beliefs about ourselves … many of these beliefs have been stored for a very long time … from childhood even … some of these beliefs and opinions are very useful and help us to *be strong and confident* … and some of them are downright harmful and destructive and have stopped us from doing many of the things we *really want to achieve* … and I believe that you would like to get rid of those destructive beliefs and create something positive inside that will make your life so much more satisfying and enjoyable.

The idea that the client's mind is *'incredibly creative and full of potential'* may be quite novel to them and should be positive and welcome

Suggests that they can change their beliefs

So … now that I mention it … I wonder if you have noticed yet that there is an entrance over there to that storehouse in your mind and the door has a sign on it 'Please come inside. You are very welcome' … I'd like you to go into the storehouse right now and look in every corner … look on every shelf … search out any mistaken or harmful belief or opinion about you or your abilities … you may want to put on some protective, confident clothing … and even a hard hat … look, it's been left for you on the shelf by your side … to protect yourself from any negative thinking you could possibly encounter. [Pause] … Good … you are now fully protected from negative thought and opinion … breathing in additional confidence with each in breath ... that's it ... have a good look around now and decide what you want to keep and what you want to throw away ... search for any mistaken belief that might have come from a former teacher ... possibly from long ago ... another child ... a family member ... a 'so called' friend ... a colleague. Sometimes people think they're being clever or funny and they call us names or give us labels and ... strangely ... we store those in our storehouse and after a while we begin to believe them ourselves ... sometimes we can even misinterpret what they originally said and we store that too ... none of those things deserves a place in your storeroom ... so please look very carefully in every corner and when you find anything that doesn't deserve to be there ... for example, some people find harmful messages that say they can't do that or they're no good at this ... (or sometimes even worse) ... if you find anything remotely like that, pick it up and chuck it into the trash can/rubbish bin/skip and nod your head when you've done it. [Pause] Good job ... don't you *feel lighter and freer now*? And certainly there must be so much more space in the storeroom now ... more room to move and experiment with new thoughts and feelings and ways of doing things ... wonderful.

Include any relevant, personal source of negativity elicited from your client

Leave plenty of time

And why not make this a space that is light and bright ... look over there and notice that there's a paintbrush and an enormous can of confident paint ... so please pick up a paintbrush and dip it in the can and paint that wonderful bright confident colour all over the walls so you can *see yourself in a new confident light*. Hey ... notice what's happening as you paint ... lots of positive messages are appearing all over the walls ... in vibrant colours and you see them clearly ... and you *read and understand them easily and well*. Look and listen ... *you are bright and you are able to learn* ... this is so important ... you are able to learn and over the next days, weeks and months you will find that you are learning an enormous variety of things ... learning to *be more confident of your ability each day* ... learning to be

Include their specific desired outcomes

267

brave enough to experiment ... *learning to recognize your strengths* and focus on these as you *develop your potential* ... *your focus and concentration is increasing* as you practise using them ... and so you find *your memory is improving and as your memory is improving and your desire to experiment becomes even stronger* ... *you will find that you are seeking out strategies to improve your reading and spelling all the time.*

And because you want to *manage your time better* ... you are learning to do it ... you are becoming even more aware of how important it is to *plan things in advance* and because you are getting better at planning ... naturally you are noticing the time more ... keeping track of it ... getting down to things more quickly. You are learning to *respect yourself for who and what you are* and *you are becoming more and more confident* all the time and ... as you have more confidence in yourself ... you know you can *deal with things resourcefully* even if they are challenging ... these are the messages and new beliefs in your storeroom now. Can you see them on the walls?

We all have to deal with challenging situations; doing it resourcefully is the key

By the way ... now you have got rid of that negativity, you no longer need that protective clothing or that hard hat ... so why don't you take them off and enjoy *absorbing all these new beliefs and messages deep inside you* ... and the wonderful thing is that in the hypnotic state of relaxation your conscious and your unconscious work particularly well together ... your unconscious will absorb all these positive ideas and your conscious mind can remind you every day to *revisit your storeroom so these beliefs will get stronger and stronger* ... helping everything to happen just as you want it to ... you can even *add to the positive beliefs on your visits* ... and whether you spend two minutes ... or twenty-two minutes ... is completely up to you ... the important thing is to *enjoy reading all the positive messages* and *refuse to allow entry to anything that could be unhelpful in any possible way.*

Both parts of the mind have their role

An ongoing means of reinforcement

So why not give yourself a moment or two to drift forward in time a few days and weeks and *notice the positive changes in you now you have begun this new habit of believing in yourself*. Can you notice the different ways … at home … at work … out and about … with people you know and people you don't know … where you *actively behave more confidently* … where you are *concentrating for longer* … where you *enjoy listening with more interest* in your eyes and ears to instructions so you understand more clearly what has to be done … at work, or wherever you are … see how *you have a calm, relaxed air about you* … believing in yourself … speaking with more authority in your voice … notice the positive look on your face … listen to the sound of your strong confident voice on the outside and your own inner voice … so much more encouraging than before … notice the positive reactions of those others around you … and best of all … see and feel how you enjoy being yourself, a really good person to be … you appreciate your life … you appreciate yourself.

Notice the useful presupposition *'now you have begun this new habit of believing in yourself'*

This section is full of positive embedded commands

VAK

Ego strengthening

Congratulations … you have begun something really wonderful here today which will *continue growing stronger and easier as each day goes by* … I think now is the time for you to begin to reorient to the room bringing back with you all your new beliefs that will have such a positive effect on your life.

A reminder that this is an ongoing process

Go to a suitable trance reorientation

Variations, Adaptations and Recommendations

This script can be adapted and used with many forms of learning differences such as dyspraxia or Asperger's syndrome. It can also be adapted for people who have physical disabilities instead of, or in addition to, learning differences. Many people have not only had to struggle with accommodating to the environment but have also had to contend with negative comments, labels and responses from peers at school or at work, from teachers, employers and sometimes even from family members which have led to low self-belief and self-esteem. Include positive suggestions relevant to their particular situations, needs and desired outcomes.

Time distortion

This short script has been adapted from *Speed up or slow down time during labour* so that it can be used for any situation where it would be useful to perceive time passing more quickly such as embarrassing, painful or invasive medical procedures, dental treatment or bearing chronic pain. It could also be appropriate for flights, other journeys or any negatively anticipated experience.

Please read the script ahead of time so you can adapt it to the needs of your client.

Interesting how *your mind can affect your body in such a positive way* ... you know how it is when we are busy or absorbed in thought ... we can *completely ignore minor aches and pains* because *we are focused on something else entirely* ... there is a part of your mind which instinctively knows when to pay attention and when *not* to pay attention to particular sensations or thoughts ... and when that part knows that *certain sensations or thoughts are of no significance at all* ... it can choose to *let them wash over you as of absolutely no significance at all ... hardly aware of them at all* ... and that part is much the same part that lets your mind *experience time in different ways* ... the time waiting for a bus in the rain may be exactly the same *clock* time as the time spent writing an email/reading a book/talking to your friend on the telephone or getting ready to go out when you're already late ... but we all know which *time seems to go faster* ... so we already have the natural ability to *speed up or slow down our perception of time at the unconscious level* and now ... in this hypnotic state ... using hypnotic thinking ... you can *strengthen that unconscious ability to perceive time differently* whenever you need to ... whenever you want to ... and so during the dental appointment/medical procedure/flight ... time *will speed up at will ... will pass more quickly* ... will *seem fairly insignificant* ... for, of course, in the totality of your life ... this time is nothing at all ... while time when *you feel well rested/calm/happy/content*

Seeds the idea of time being perceived differently according to our focus of attention

Suggests that the ability to speed up or slow down perceived time is natural and that this ability can be enhanced through the hypnotic thinking

Negative experiences can pass more quickly

271

will slow down and you can really *enjoy those confident/calm/comfortable feelings* for so much longer ... and *you tend to be very aware of each moment of that time ... taking an active pleasure in it* ... you *notice how positive you feel* ... and possibly even people around you will seem to notice and comment on how good you look ... how well you are handling any situation.

Happy times can be expanded

So why not take a little time now ... which might seem like a long time ... *to see yourself in your mind's eye, how things are going so well for you* ... see how you are dealing with everything so well while you are so focused on some positive thought ... your mind has learned its lesson very well without even consciously thinking how it did it ... *it's speeding up any possible uncomfortable time/tricky situation/time in the dental surgery/time in the hospital/ flight time so you are coping with it easily and calmly* ... *you can bear any tricky/difficult/uncomfortable situation/circumstances with great equanimity because you know it/they will pass quickly* ... that's right ... your unconscious mind is reminding you that *you can derive a great deal of satisfaction from being able to let any chosen time pass more quickly* ... and ... even better ... your mind will also do something else amazing ... *it will slow down every minute of comfortable/positive/enjoyable time so you can notice yourself noticing* the feeling of comfort/enjoyment/enthusiasm/contentment ... and when you look back ... and you will do ... you may well feel a sense of pride through knowing that you *were able to take everything in your stride at this very special time*. It's also good to remember *that* ... although you will retain an ability to deliberately perceive time differently in situations where it would be appropriate ... your everyday perception of time will of course return to normal in every way.

Add specific relevant suggestions. Have them visualise carrying out their desired outcome calmly and confidently

Reminder that their perception of time will return to normal

Go to a suitable trance reorientation or add in further appropriate suggestions

Positive thinking

For either personal or workplace settings.

Many years ago on holiday when I was travelling from San Francisco up to Seattle I was involved in a car crash as a passenger and … although not seriously hurt … was badly shaken up and … when we resumed our journey, with a new hire car, two or three days later … found I was trembling, with tears of fear running down my cheeks each time a car approached on the other side of the road, and this continued for at least a day or two … until there came a moment when I had a sudden realisation of what I was really doing … I was the one who was now ruining my holiday and my husband's holiday too. Of course … *originally* … the truck that ploughed into us had wrecked the car and lost us two or three days of our trip but … after resuming our journey … I was the only one responsible for sabotaging our enjoyment … I was the one who was achieving nothing but causing misery to myself and unease to the driver … my fear couldn't have helped in any way whatsoever … even in an emergency my fear would probably have made things worse … I had a sudden moment of clarity … in fact, it was life-changing … I realised that I *had the power to stop it* … I had the power to *stop this negative thinking* … I had the power to *take control of my thoughts rather than let the thoughts be in control of me* and … strange though this may seem … suddenly it came to me … suddenly I thought, *'actually it's easy'* … so I made my choice … I would just *stop thinking of everything bad that could happen* and instead I would *think of positive things that could happen* and, in fact, that's exactly what I did … I discovered that I could *enjoy the moment* … I discovered that I had the power to *let myself enjoy the wonderful scenery* as we drove up the coastal road … *appreciate the blue of the sky and the changing colours of the sea and be pleased and grateful to be alive.*

You can 'borrow' my very real experience here or you can substitute some similar mind-changing experience of your own

Embedded commands to the client within the framework of a personal anecdote about you

Encourage the imagination of positive colours and scenery as a backdrop to change

And from that moment, I decided to change my outlook in general … not only about the chance of an accident … I found a way to *make the most of the moment* … I would *notice the positive and focus on that* … and you know … if *you actually truly want to* … *you can do that too* … *here and now* … *you have the power to stop negative thinking* … *you have the power* … you can *make a decision to put a positive slant on what you encounter in your life* … *it is absolutely your prerogative to view things from a positive perspective when that is what you want to do* … *come to any situation with an open mind* and … when you think about it … doesn't it generally make more sense to *adopt a more positive outlook where you can (?)*… now, of course, I'm not trying to say that bad things don't happen or that negatives don't exist because you and I both know that they do sometimes happen, but what I *am saying* is that … when you *approach the majority of situations with a positive outlook and an intention to find something useful or interesting* … *life is generally more enjoyable for you* … *and life is certainly more enjoyable for those around you* … optimism and enthusiasm are quite catching … and quite uplifting too.

Ostensibly talking about oneself, there are opportunities to slip in embedded commands

Here it moves to talking directly about the client, suggesting that they also have the power to change

Points out that adopting a more positive approach can help cope more effectively with negative events

Now the fact is … we know that the reason you're here today is because your old habit of focusing on the negative has been weighing you down and hindering you in both your working and home life … you thought it would be useful for you to *feel more positive about things* … *let go of that old way* … *and* … *in the end* … *it all comes down to one decision* … so I'm wondering if *you are really prepared to make that decision now* … and *give yourself the opportunity of doing something different for a while* … so that you can *compare the feelings* … *compare the difference in approach* … *compare the results of looking for a positive in a situation with the results of your old focus on a negative outcome* … you could for example decide to *adopt a more optimistic strategy* for a week/two weeks/a month and notice the differences that makes to you … to others too

Reminding the client of their purpose in being with you

It is sensible to arrange a follow up appointment in 'a week/two weeks/a month' to discover feedback and reinforce motivation

... do it as a kind of experiment ... you could even keep a notebook and *write down the interesting differences you notice* so when you look back, you can remember the little details that have changed in your outlook ... and then only because you want to ... and only because *you really want to* ... you can decide to *stick with your more positive outlook* on life because you have the power ... yes, you really do have the power ... to *just do it right* ... *do it right now for you*. Great ... let me know once you have made this decision. [Pause]

Presupposition *'you really want to'*

Presupposes the decision will be made

Let's take a few moments to check this out with the part of you that always used to seek out the negative aspects of things ... explain to this part of you ... mentally and silently ... that you understand it probably had a rationale for doing this ... probably it had some sense of forewarning you of potential disaster or protecting you from disappointment ... but the net result of it was ... contrary to what it really had in mind for you ... actually to cause you problems rather than to protect you from them ... (perhaps even to hold you back/depress you ... maybe depress other people too). Tell it that you appreciate what it was trying to do for you but explain that actually now you want to experiment and *try out a different way of dealing with life* for a given period of time ... this way will consist of looking for the positive in a scenario before assuming it doesn't exist. Ask that part for its help for an agreed period of time ... as an experiment ... with a review in two weeks/four weeks ... and then let me know when you have its agreement. [Pause] Very good.

Parts reframe

(Should there be no agreement, suggest that you are about to explain a very important new role for it to play)

Excellent ... please ask the part if it will accept a new and very important role ... this role is to *remind you of all your inner strengths and resources* any and every time a possible difficulty might arise ...also to remind you of previous times and occasions where *you have been able to cope with events ... cope with people ... cope with inner feelings supremely well.* In this way you can *expect to feel well prepared*

Give the part a different and positive role to play

A way to include embedded commands within a suggestion to speak or negotiate with a part

*to deal with anybody ... respond calmly and confi-
dently to any internal or external feeling ... even deal
with disappointments with a sense of strength and
optimism which will be far more empowering than
before.* Please do that now and let me know when
*you have the agreement of your unconscious and
are ready to move on and zoom forward in time to
observe some of the positive results of your change
of approach.* [Pause]

'***when** you have*' not '**if** *you
have*'

So, very good ... now is the time to have a look at
the results of that empowering decision to *change
your focus ...* I invite you to run a mental film of your
everyday life at home ... at work ... in any situation
where *your decision today will have influenced your
thinking ... your feeling and your way of behaving ...*
and take some time to explore how *these changes in
you will be benefitting not only yourself but all those
people around you ...* and I'd also like you to notice
... because of the reminders from that protective
part of you ... that *you are becoming more aware
of your strengths and abilities* ... and ... rather than
being downcast when things don't go according
to plan ... it seems that *you are becoming more
resourceful in finding ways around things ...* looking
for solutions ... there's almost an excitement as you
seek out opportunities to *create something positive ...* is it that *you have become more proactive
and less reactive*? [Pause] Excellent ... can you run
over the best parts again this time being particularly
aware of what you see ... the feelings inside ... any
inner words of encouragement ... any comments
from others that let you know that other people are
benefitting from your change of outlook ... take all
the time *you want to do that* and let me know when
you've done so. [Pause] Well done.

'Forward pace' the
changes

Presupposition

Embedded commands

Repetition reinforces the
effect

VAK

Allow all the time they
need

Now all of this seems so rewarding that I am sure
that you will want to *keep the positive change in
you ...* and ... you will remember to *keep to your
commitment to review your results in two weeks/
four weeks from now ...* maybe you will want to

make some adjustments so that *every part of you feels valued and fully involved in this ... every part of you involved in giving you a better quality of life ...* I believe it's just about time for you to begin reorienting to the room ... and ... as you do ... I'm wondering just where and how *you are already experiencing a sense of excitement and curiosity about the next few days and weeks.*

Go to a suitable trance reorientation

Variations, Adaptations and Recommendations

This script would be very suitable for use in a workplace coaching environment as well as in the hypnotherapy office/consulting room.

After reorientation from the trance, it would be useful to reinforce the client's commitment to review the changes achieved after the agreed period of time. This will keep all parts on board with the new positive approach, which, during the trance, was negotiated as a time-limited experiment. This review could be purely internal and need not involve another appointment, although this would of course provide further reinforcement. In the workplace coaching environment, setting a review date would seem to be normal procedure.

The script has been designed for use in a content-free manner so that the therapist avoids becoming overinvolved in the content and can use his or her skills to guide the client through the mental process itself, remembering to allow plenty of time for reflective thought. However, if appropriate, it can easily be adapted and used in a more interactive question and answer style.

Finding mislaid items

Although this is a generic script suitable for locating any mislaid item, I have used the specific scenario of mislaid jewellery in this script for the purposes of illustration. Mislaid jewellery seems to be a common problem, and I have been asked to assist many clients in this regard over the years. Replace the shaded areas of text with examples from your client's own situation. Get answers to your questions as you go along because occasionally people only recall the memory in the trance state and forget it once they reorient to the non-hypnotic state.

Relaxing so comfortably and focusing on the sound of my voice can *give you a wonderful experience here today of comfort and ease* … comfort and ease all the way through your body … and comfort and ease all through your mind … and have you ever noticed just *how much easier it is to daydream when you feel comfortable and at ease*? There's nothing that you have to do except *enjoy drifting and dreaming* … when you dream … I wonder if you … like me … ever have those *dreams that are sometimes so vivid* that you can hardly believe they are not real? They are so vivid and realistic that sometimes when I wake, it takes a few moments for me to decide if it was really only a dream since all the pictures in my mind were so clear … so bright … so real … every detail so vivid … I *really enjoy those dreams.*

> Invites revivification of the client's shared similar dream experiences. Even if they haven't had such an experience they will benefit from the commands embedded in the text

I wonder how quickly you'll be surprised to **discover** that … as you *drift and dream* you also have the strange … almost contradictory experience … of **a clear focus on every important item** in your dream … that's the interesting thing about dreams … dreams are often contradictory but contain **hidden meanings and truths that shine through** when you *allow them to do so* … **every hidden thing** seems to **become clear and obvious in your mind** and maybe you'll **enjoy becoming aware of** inner thoughts and **memories** sometimes long since forgotten … memories from long ago … and more recently too … which will **delight you as**

> Words in bold should be given extra emphasis since they contain a subtext to enhance the memory

you recall them *... missing links occur* while you **dream here ...** and later too ... *and* **will pop into your mind now** *or indeed* when you're least expecting them ... when you're thinking about something else entirely ... *just a* **surprising reminder** *that makes* **everything fit together** ... *a bit like one of those Eureka moments ... you know ... when you think to yourself* **'I've got it!' or 'I know it.'**

So would you now be willing to *experience a sense of heightened awareness* as you *enjoy going deeper into this relaxing daydream* ... and let yourself *become more and more aware of sensations of calm and comfort* spreading around your body? Noticing too ... inner thoughts and feelings that had been forgotten in the mists of time ... *drifting up through those hazy mists into the clear light of day* ... the more you *relax now*, *the more crystal clear your thoughts become* ... going deeper and deeper into that amazing state where all *your mental processes become enhanced* ... the clarity of thought ... the ability to see things in your mind's eye ... the ability to recall events, voices, feelings with an immediacy that surprises and delights.

Several embedded commands occur within the one question, all encouraging recall and clarity of thought

You know, *we all have an amazing capacity to remember things more easily than we think* ... even those people who say they don't *have very good memories* ... because everyone can remember things when they're in the right relaxed frame of mind ... everyone has the ability to *remember events just as if they happened yesterday* ... think about it ... when we let ourselves *go right back into a memory* ... we can feel a particular emotion, for example ... just as if it were happening today at this very moment ... we do it all the time to *remember positive feelings* of happy occasions ... and sometimes it makes us smile or laugh while we *remember the detail* ... or have you ever had that experience of going to a room for a purpose and when you got there you couldn't remember why you went? And then you go back to the place when you made the

This section contains a mixture of reframes and truisms about memory, helping to convince the client of their ability to remember well

An example of the role of emotion in memory

Embedded command to *'remember the detail'*

decision to do that thing in the first place ... *and it all comes back to you so easily* ... you just needed the place/the context to *stimulate the memory* and then you were able to *find the memory quite naturally and easily.*

An example of context dependent memory

You can choose to do the next part from a dissociated (detached) point of view by asking the client to float up above the situation and look down on it as if watching a movie

Or you can get them to adopt an associated view as if they are completely reliving the situation in the present moment

Or you can first ask them to look from a dissociated point of view and then 'drop down' into the memory, thus taking advantage of both perspectives

Or you can just ask them to float back into the memory and allow them to do whatever comes most naturally to them

So you are in the perfect frame of mind now ... the hypnotic frame of mind ... to *recall things quite effortlessly ... recall every detail with enhanced clarity of vision* ... so why not now let your mind drift right back into that time where you are completely sure in your mind that you saw that ring ... that's it ... and looking at it now in your mind's eye, tell me where you are and where the ring is. [Pause and await their answer] So, you're in the bedroom ... and as you look at the ring on your finger now, notice some of the other things in the room ... what can you see? [Pause and await their answer] What can you hear? [Pause and await their answer] Notice your thoughts ... what are you thinking about? [Pause and await their answer] How are you feeling? [Pause and await their answer] What are you doing now? [Pause and await their answer]

More suggestions for enhanced memory

Use the present tense to encourage a sense of reliving the situation in the present moment. Give plenty of time for them to reflect before answering your questions

The reason for asking about thoughts and feelings is to stimulate context or state dependent memories of subsequent actions

So you're looking in the mirror ... look at your fingers ... tell me what you can see ... [Pause and await their answer] You can see the ring is still on your finger ... what are you thinking as you look in the mirror? ... [Pause and await their answer] Ah, you notice that your nails are long and you need to look for a nail file ... are you doing that now? [Pause and

Continue moving through their memory of events with prompts and questions. You can use devices such as fast forward, rewind, a zoom lens for more detail, stepping back for the bigger picture, shining spotlights on dark areas

await their answer] Where are you looking? [Pause and await their answer] What are you thinking? [Pause and await their answer] OK. As you <u>open that drawer, notice that you have a very bright torch and shine it into the drawer as you look inside</u> ... what do you see? [Pause and await their answer]

If they recall the information, simply congratulate their unconscious mind for the good work and go straight to a trance reorientation with suggestions to be completely back in the present moment as they reorient to their surroundings

And today you have begun an unconscious search for information which will *continue now at the innermost level* while you just get on with your life in the normal way ... *your unconscious will continue sifting through files of information and when it uncovers something interesting it will bring it to the attention of your conscious mind* ... this often happens when you are absorbed in something else entirely ... or even in your dreams as you sleep and, when you wake in the morning, that interesting information may be waiting there for you ... so don't be too surprised when *memories occur to you* at very odd times and places ... usually sooner ... occasionally later ... than you think ... as you *consciously and patiently get on with your everyday life and your unconscious gets on with its journey of discovery.*

If they have not recalled the information at this point, give suggestions for information to occur to them at any time over the upcoming days

Go to a suitable trance reorientation with suggestions to be completely back in the present moment as they reorient to their surroundings

Habits

Letting go of habits – generic template for nail biting

The underscored areas refer to nail biting and can be replaced with words and phrases relevant to the habit you are addressing. A very similar framework has been used in *Let go of panic*.

The use of a progressive relaxation, or a hand levitation induction in the case of nail biting, would be appropriate.

Just listening and relaxing and accepting positive suggestions that will help you *achieve your aim/ objective/whatever you want to achieve* for your overall well-being now you have made the decision to *let go of that old unhelpful habit* of nail biting/ picking/chewing/sucking your fingers ... all you need to do is to *enjoy just listening and relaxing and accepting the positive suggestions* of your own choosing that we discussed and as you *go deeper and deeper* you *enjoy even more just listening and relaxing* ... just enjoying accepting the positive suggestions of your own choosing which will *improve your appearance immeasurably ... improve your self esteem immeasurably* ... just listening and relaxing ... that's it ... paying more and more attention to the sound of my voice ... understanding how much you really want to have nice hands/well groomed hands/ longer, stronger nails/comfortable smooth fingertips ... just listening and relaxing and accepting my voice as you *go deeper and deeper relaxed* ... hear *my voice soothing you with each suggestion you accept* as you go even deeper and deeper ... just listening and *enjoying accepting* this gift ... *feel yourself accepting* that at last *you are changing things to your advantage* ... it's something you've wanted for so long and *now you can have it* ... it's yours as you *go into the deepest trance ever* ... knowing now there is no going back on your decision and being so grateful for that ... accepting more and more ... almost completely there now as you listen .... just listening and accepting and becoming more and

Using a rhythmic delivery within a 'stream of consciousness' approach works well with this script

The presupposition 'you have made the decision' is followed by the embedded command 'to *let go of that old unhelpful habit*'

Sounds like a long awaited gift to be accepted

more completely relaxed … so *completely sure you are doing the right thing* … so deep and accepting … hearing and *feeling the truth of my voice now* … feel my words that you *can't wait to accept them* and you *feel drawn to follow them* … you *feel compelled to follow them* … *following every word* … *following every single step of the way* … you're going to find that the old unwanted picking/biting behaviour is starting to slip/*drift away from your mind as you go deeper and deeper* … *drift away from your body/fingers* as you go deeper and deeper … *drift away from your being all together* as you go deeper and deeper …you are more and more sure that the old behaviour has been drifting away as though it has nothing to do with you now … no longer a part of you … almost as though *it was never there* and it will *become more and more difficult to* bring it to mind no matter how hard you might try … and the harder you tried the more difficult it would become … in truth *you are delighted that the* new behaviour/habit/calm way of doing things *is becoming more and more what you want for you* … your impulses are changing as you are just enjoying listening and relaxing and accepting that a need for nice smooth skin on your fingers is growing stronger as your nails are growing stronger … the new behaviour is drifting into you … is embedding itself into you … as part of you … it's what you really want … your desire to keep your nails and hands smooth will grow stronger and stronger as each day it is becoming more and more part of your own inner way of thinking … more and more part of your own inner way of behaving … it becomes more of a need than a desire … more of a compulsion … inner level and outer level … more and more part of you … your confidence is growing daily … here and now as you are going deeper and deeper still … your belief in you is settling in deeper and deeper … growing stronger and stronger … your belief in your confidence and your ability to do things calmly and confidently without recourse to those old ways … your belief in you is growing stronger and stronger … the old habit has been

Reassuring to be told 'you are doing the right thing'

'can't wait to accept' **and** 'you *feel compelled*' **are difficult to resist**

The law of reversed effect

'embedding itself into you' **If something is 'embedded' it is difficult to dislodge**

'settling in deeper and deeper' ***Once again this seems difficult to dislodge***

disappearing and you are feeling more and more at one with your new habit which suits you better ... more and more comfortable and at ease with it ... more and more confident and comfortable in the new habit being part of you ... in fact so comfortable and so confident that it hardly seems like a new habit at all ... it just seems what you do ... and ... of course ... what you *avoid* doing ... you love being 'this you' with this way of doing things ... it's so right for you ... this is the way things are ... this is your normality now ... you find you are thinking calmly and confidently ... happy and content in the way you do things now ... knowing that everything seems right now ... more appropriate now ... more 'you' now ... no need for self recriminations any longer ... just a need to keep the changes now at the inner level and the outer level and all the way though ... You think calmly and confidently ... you feel calm and confident you behave calmly and confidently so you find that any old perceived need for those unhelpful/harmful/unpleasant/childish/unattractive actions have simply faded away ... have disappeared completely ... what a wonderful relief.

So just before you reorient to the room I'd like you to look ahead in your mind to four weeks from now when your new way of doing things has been completely internalised ... and notice how it has also been externalised ... look at you so much calmer in those old situations where you used to get stressed ... notice that your hands are in your lap/by your sides/holding those papers/anywhere but near your mouth/and look more closely and see how they look so much more attractive/neat/tidy/well groomed than they used to be ... you are doing whatever you need to do to keep them that way ... filing/manicuring your nails and every time you have done this has reinforced this need/desire you have to keep them nice ... see how you are glancing down at your hands from time to time ... can't resist a little smile of satisfaction ... taking a pride in what you see ...

Personalise this guided visualization of a successful outcome with pre-elicited information

feel the difference … I wonder who has noticed how <u>well-kept your nails are now</u> and that the impression you give is so much more <u>business-like/personable/ calm/confident</u> … because of course the difference is not only that <u>your appearance is so much more groomed</u> … it is that *you are so much more content and satisfied with yourself on the inside and determined to do whatever you need to do to ensure that all of this continues … internally and externally.*

Other people noticing and commenting on a new behaviour is thought to reinforce it

Go to a trance reorientation. Where a hand levitation induction has been used, remember to remove any suggestions of inappropriate sensations induced in the trance state

Variations, Adaptations and Recommendations

This script can be adapted for use with other habits/anxious responses such as fiddling and twiddling hair, blushing or thumb-sucking (yes, some adults still do it!).

Some problems may be best dealt with by first addressing the original cause, but there may still be elements that persist which are habitual in nature. This script may be adapted and used successfully in these cases too. An automatic irritable response, procrastination, negative thinking, OCD responses and even smoking and comfort eating have responded well to this approach used as part of an overall treatment strategy.

Delete unwanted habits/compulsive behaviour and reprogram thinking

This script can be adapted for use with almost any habit, obsessive or compulsive behaviour. It is presented here in its simplest form but can be extended in many different ways as suggested in the Variations at the end of the script.

These days most of us are very familiar with using computer technology whether through PCs or lap-tops or net books or phones so it's probably a very natural way to think about the mind ... and actually ... the mind is far and away superior in being able to run programs for the body ... for language ... for emotions ... for our psychological well-being ... for storing habits ... and for every aspect of our lives really.

Truism

Now you've been talking about that habit of putting everything in a special order and a feeling of 'having' to have everything in a very particular place and 'needing' to rearrange it exactly as it was, if it becomes disturbed in any way ... now it's useful to know that there is a program that runs your habits ... so can you just go into your mental computer and look for that icon and let me know once you've clicked on it ... Great.

Now click on Options and you'll find 'Attitudes' ... and when you click on that you will find two choices ... '*I want to change*' and 'I don't want to change' so click on the one you want and tell me what it is ... [Their response: 'I want to change'] Great ... you want to change ... now you will notice a Settings Option for how much you want to *make that change* on a scale of 1–10 ... please have a look at these and consider where you are on that scale ... you may want to adjust it perhaps?

If no positive response, you will need to re-examine objectives and fears and then reframe

Now ... you need to have a look at what's been going wrong with the program ... so, can you go into it and check for any thinking errors ... find what's flagged up there … you might see something like 'you have to arrange everything in order/you have to check everything three times before you can be certain' … when you find an error like this, please can you go in and firmly delete it as it has no right to be in that program at all … excellent … keep searching and only stop and let me know once you have deleted them all. [Pause] Well done.

So of course now you need to program positive thoughts and instructions to ensure that you carry out everything in a way that is so much more appropriate/in keeping with your wishes/more helpful so how about clicking on the positive beliefs icon and type in … I can take control of my thoughts … even if an old habitual thought begins, I can take control and reject it … I am stronger than I used to think I was … I refused to be controlled or intimidated by faulty ideas, I can take control of my own thinking … I can stand up to mistaken messages … I will automatically delete error messages as soon as they occur … Please click on save and just take a moment to congratulate yourself on a job well done.

Excellent work … I am sure you would enjoy previewing the results of your work here today … so please click on the Preview Icon to see the program in action … good … see yourself there in your house where your new program is running perfectly … what is it about you that lets you know things have changed so radically? How do you look? How do you feel inside? Look into your mind and listen to your thoughts … what is it that lets you know how they are so much more positive now? … Are other people noticing yet the differences in you or is it just you that feels so much better? Now run through any other scenarios where there are changes to be noticed … at work for example … or socialising … and once you have seen all you need to see for today … you can do one final thing … go to the attitudes and settings option once more and check that your 'I want to change' settings are exactly where

Mention any faulty thinking patterns you have elicited beforehand

Presupposition

Select any appropriate messages from these and include any others specific to your particular client

Presupposition

Future pace

Presuppositions of change

VAK

Notice the effect of the word 'yet' in 'noticing *yet* the differences'

you need them to be for optimum results and save everything. Fantastic.

Time in a moment for you to begin that process of reorientation to alert awareness of how vey good you feel and how reassuring it is to know that *your unconscious mind will be monitoring and adjusting all systems over the forthcoming days and weeks to ensure continued progress and successful results.*

Go to a suitable trance reorientation

Variations, Adaptations and Recommendations

This metaphor can be extended in various ways as appropriate to the problem and the individual client.

FLAG UP ERROR MESSAGE

This can be set to flag up any error in thinking with a big red sign in the mind every time it occurs with a command to ignore/delete the thought and choose an alternative behaviour.

PREVIEW BEHAVIOUR SCREEN IN 'SAFE MODE'

If a compulsive or obsessive behaviour is so strong that it would be inconceivable initially for the client to attempt to lose it completely, they could use a coping behaviour as a first step towards eventual eradication of the habit. The mental rehearsal of this first step could be carried out using the analogy of running the computer in 'safe mode'. This could be used over a number of sessions with increasing progress until such time as they feel able to preview the final desired behaviour change using the preview screen in 'normal mode'.

OPTIONS MENU

This can be used to accommodate any additional reframing of choices, changes in belief or extra resources needed using typical menu options, for example Format, Edit, Insert, Tools.

VIRUS CHECKER

Run the scan and apply suitable fixes.

FAULTY THINKING PATTERNS

Typical thinking patterns underlie obsessive thoughts and behaviours, for example, those listed below. Research cognitive behaviour therapy approaches for more detail. The computer analogy can be employed to type in more accurate or acceptable beliefs:

- Over estimating the importance of a thought
- Over estimating the possibility of a danger
- A feeling of responsibility for events beyond their control
- Perfectionism and over strict standards
- Finding it difficult to tolerate ambiguous situations
- Feeling that anxiety is difficult or impossible to tolerate.

Inductions and Deepeners

Comfort

This also appears in the script *Change anxious thoughts*.

And as you sit there, you can become aware of any possible stored tensions that you'd like to let go ... and ... just as soon as you're ready ... you can choose to *let them go with your breathing* ... and this may be the time ... when you need to *let yourself begin to find a way to rest right now* ... building your calm ... and *do know that you have that calm and confidence* deep down within you ... settling yourself down ... calm and confidence drifting up to the surface ... so I'd like you at first to *let only your eyelids rest* now ... letting every tiny little muscle and nerve ending rest and let go, don't worry about the *rest* of you ... just concentrate on letting your eyelids *rest* ... that's right, making them more comfortable now, let the feeling of comfort *spread right through the eyes, feel the comfort* and *know it's safe to enjoy those feelings of comfort now* ... and as you listen to the sound of the voice and as a calm feeling is beginning to come upon you ... so you can *begin to feel the comfort spreading* further ... and every place that it touches in your mind and body can *notice that comfort spreading calm* ... and now your eyelids are *really* resting, can you notice that different parts of your body are beginning to *feel more comfortable now?* And it's good to let them *feel even more comfortable now* ... *all over* ... *all the way through.*

'and this may be the time' **is deliberately ambiguous as it relates both to the phrases before and after it**

Juxtaposition of 'settling down' **and** 'calm and confidence drifting up'

'let *only* your eyelids rest now' **removes any potential worries of not being able to relax**

The word 'safe' **is reassuring and the sentence links ideas of safety, listening, calm and comfort together**

Now come the suggestions of calm spreading to other parts of the body

Mental massage

This induction is highly recommended where you wish your client to achieve a deep level of relaxation, for example with conditions such as IBS.

Make yourself comfortable and ... in your own time ... allow your eyelids to close so that you can *enjoy an experience of relaxation* and whether you *experience this relaxation deeply* ... or lightly ... it's a time when you can ... do something just for you ... nobody else but you ... do something to help you *feel more comfortable now* ... *all over* ... *all the way through* ... just listening to the sound of my voice ... and begin ... very, very gently ... a process of calming relaxation ... *enjoy an experience of internal comfort* ... where there is no right way and no wrong way to *experience this sense right away* ... of your thoughts drifting ... your thoughts drifting off to no special place ... or maybe some special calming place ... maybe somewhere you know ... maybe some quiet, calm place in you ... a place of calm awareness in you of what *you really want calm in your life* ... *calm and comfort in your tummy/belly/ stomach/body.*

'no right way and no wrong way' removes any pressure

Intentional running of one phrase into another to bypass the conscious mind

And know you can ... truly *enjoy those feelings of comfort* ... *fully* ... *very soon* ... it's safe ... to drift and just listen to the sound of the voice ... and as you listen to the sound of the voice ... you may perhaps be aware of other sounds inside or outside the room ... and it may surprise you ... or it may *seem perfectly natural* ... that these sounds don't bother you at all ... they don't disturb you at all ... they may even *reassure you* ... so you can *drift into even deeper* ... more comfortable ... feelings of ease and relaxation ... and as you *notice the pause* ... between the words ... the pause can remind you ... it's ... *time for you to pause too* ... *pause to relax* ... *pause to do nothing* ... and yet ... *do something* ... *very important for you* ... pause to *take time out* ... just as people take time out of a

Manipulation of sounds to fade away or act as triggers of deeper relaxation

busy life for a massage …time to *relax your body … relax your mind … release any possible tension* with your breathing … enjoy a sense of healing hands massaging all the tension away from every part of the body.

Seeds the idea of massage

And some people describe hypnotic relaxation as being just like a mental massage … which I think is a lovely idea … you can *try it out now* … so you can tell me later *how well this idea fits with you* … so perhaps you could begin by letting all the tiny little muscles in your eyelids *relax even more than before* … that's it … let them really, really relax … let them go completely droopy, drowsy, dreamy, … that's right … become aware of how … just by letting your eyelids relax completely … it seems to set up a chain reaction where those wonderful, comfortable relaxed feelings spread from one set of muscles into another … all on their own … in fact … I wonder whether you have already noticed how those comfortable feelings have been spreading into your cheeks … around your nose … around your mouth … (if you've ever had a facial massage you may recognize the feelings) … into your jaw … into your neck … yes … *let all those muscles go* droopy, drowsy, dreamy … that's it … that's right … just let all the muscles … *relax* … the muscles in the back of your head … *relax* … let all the tiny little muscles in the scalp … relax … that's good … really good … the tiny little muscles in your scalp relaxing just as though … somehow … your own fingers … could … massage your muscles … easing the tension … relaxing. … Are they your own fingers? … Or are they expert masseur's fingers … kneading your shoulders? Easing out the tension … letting all the muscles in your shoulders relax … *comfort and ease spreading all through the shoulders* … spreading down from the shoulders and into the arms … massaging any tension out of the muscles … out of the tissues … massaging all the way down through the arms … and down through the elbows … down into the hands and the fingers

Now, a 'mental' massage

Alliteration is always effective

For many people 'a facial massage' will revivify calm, relaxing feelings

'your own fingers' are very non-threatening

Or, maybe they prefer the idea of 'an expert's fingers'

... that's right ... all the tension flowing out through the fingertips. ... Great job.

And have you noticed that now your shoulders are so much more relaxed ... those comfortable feelings have been spreading into your back ... feeling the muscles being massaged all around your back ... relax ... let all the muscles relax in your back ... relax your upper back ... the fingers relaxing the muscles all the way down your spine ... relax your lower back ... all through the trunk of your body ... into your lower body ... into your thighs ... just let all those muscles go ... that's it ... that's right ... just let all the tension flow down through the legs ... down through the knees ... down through the lower legs ... relaxing all the muscles ... feeling the ease spreading all the way down ... any tension flowing down through the feet ... and continuing down into and out ... right out ... of the very tips of your toes.

The massage continues

And can you *notice now* ... *really* notice ... how ... as all of those wonderful feelings of comfort and calm have been spreading through the body ... every single *internal* organ has been relaxing too ... on the inside ... all the way through ... the amazing feeling of pure relaxation seems to spread all through the muscles and nerves in your entire body ... interesting to experience how you are ... at one and the same time ... aware that you are so relaxed and yet hardly aware of your body at all.

'really notice' **suggests a need to look more closely**

The stress on *'internal'* **organs suggests an even deeper level of relaxation and is of course particularly useful to precede a script dealing with IBS**

The lift or elevator

This is a particularly suitable induction for use in the workplace where the focus is more on coaching than on therapy since it can be carried out in a purely conversational way with no mention of hypnosis. It can be suggested as a technique just to focus attention although undoubtedly it will induce a light state of trance. Clearly this would not be a suitable induction for anyone suffering with claustrophobia or phobias of lifts/elevators.

Maybe you'd like to (put your pen down and just) sit comfortably and focus your attention on that paperweight/pen holder/light switch as you take a moment or two to *clarify your thinking … clear your mind of extraneous thoughts …* and *notice how soon …* as *your vision blurs …* or … strangely … as the outlines even seem to have become intensely defined … *your eyelids seem to have an irresistible urge to blink …* or *close …* which is absolutely fine … it just means that *your mind is so ready to focus on what is important here today* that it wants to *cut out all forms of distractions …* that's right … and *become quite creative in your thinking.*

Vision blurs or outlines intensify as a natural result of intense focus, and a natural urge to blink will ensue

Imbues a natural response 'an urge to blink' with a meaning, e.g. *'your mind is so ready to focus'*

So … quite creatively … I'd like you to imagine that you are waiting outside the lift/elevator to go up to the top floor to a very important meeting … your eyes are following the signs/lights signalling its approach towards your floor … the chime/sound announces its arrival and the doors open … you step inside, press the button for the top floor and, as the doors close, your eyes will quite naturally *turn to the visual display …* that's it … as the lift/elevator rises … can you *notice how you become more and more focused* as you pass through each floor? … *Your clarity of thought increases and intensifies* as the numbers change … perhaps you begin to *be more aware of different perspectives?* … Do you begin to *feel more open to new possibilities?* … Perhaps wanting to invite others' opinions … *really* listening and discussing ideas with an open mind? … And as you *feel that sensation in your body …*

Use your voice to emphasise the embedded commands in the questions just before you arrive at your floor … can *you sense that surge of excitement* when the doors open and you walk out? … There will be new insights/new opportunities/interesting explorations/changes and decisions to be made. [Pause] Look … the doors are opening … only walk out when *you're ready to explore/continue/experience something interesting that will improve your life immeasurably … and let me know/nod your head when you're ready.*

'Yes set' questions and statements

These 'pre' induction questions form a mini induction of their own. They are, of course, based on Milton Erickson's idea of a set of questions designed to secure agreement and therefore a positive mindset as a person drifts into the trance state. Use a light, questioning tone of voice throughout.

So ... we've spoken about what the problem is ... how, when and where it happens ... we've spoken about what makes it worse ... and what makes it better, have we not?

Just checking now that I'm right in thinking that there's nothing more that you want to add before we *move on to the next stage*? Is that so?

And *you are really sure that the time has come* for you to do something now to sort this out/crack this/ deal with this/put an end to this/put this behind you once and for all?

And you're certain, are you not, that I've answered all your questions about the state of hypnotic relaxation that is known as trance?

And are you ready now to *increase your level of physical comfort and relaxation* so that you can *receive the positive suggestions in the nicest possible way*?

And you know, don't you, that if you want to move around at any time to *increase your physical comfort,* you are more than free to do so?

And you are aware, aren't you, that you can relax just as lightly or just as deeply as you want?

And as you begin now to *sense a pleasant feeling of relaxation spreading over you* ... you can enjoy going just as deeply as is comfortable for you to *make the most of all the positive ideas that you consider are just right for you.*

The questions and statements are designed to secure mental agreement of the client, whether silent or spoken. The questions assume that the client has already been assured of these points, but if not, they will act as reassurance in themselves

You can continue in this vein until the client has drifted into an appropriate state of trance or you can move into another induction or deepener

Ratio breathing

This can be used as an induction or a deepener and also appears in the *Anxiety, Panic, Phobias* section as a calming activity in its own right.

Settle yourself comfortably in the chair and let your eyes close and begin to imagine that the air around you is a wonderful colour of calm and comfort ... I wonder what colour that would be ... and as I count from 1 to 3 ... I'd like you to breathe in through your nose that wonderful calming, comforting colour so it spreads through your whole body ... are you ready? ... In 2, 3 ... Out 2, 3, 4, 5, 6 ... In 2, 3 ... Out 2, 3, 4, 5, 6 ... and *each time you breathe out through your nose, you can breathe out any tension in your body* ... you can even look inside and notice the colour of that tension and ... as we count out ... just breathe out that colour ... Out 2, 3, 4, 5, 6 ... *breathe away any tension in your mind* ... that's right .... breathing In 2, 3 ... Out 2, 3, 4, 5, 6 ... In 2, 3 ... Out 2, 3, 4, 5, 6 ... and *each time you do this ... your level of calm and comfort increases* ... you *become more and more relaxed ... you become more and more in control of your relaxation* ... and this *will continue as we go on.*

So ... as you've been breathing in the calm to the count of three and breathing out the tension to the count of six ... have you been noticing just *how very calming this is?* ... How it *gives you control over your breathing and control over your feelings* ... and every time you do this ... always remembering to *breathe only through your nose* ... you will strengthen your ability to *stay calm and in control in any situation* ... you have a tool you can use anywhere ... any time ... you want to *increase your calm and increase your control.* So in a moment or two I'm going to begin the counting again and then I'm going to allow you to continue your own inner counting ... keeping the rhythm ... breathing in through your nose and out through your nose ... breathing in the calm ... and

This script makes use of the simple controlled breathing technique where you breathe in to the count of 3 and out to the count of 6, or in to the count of 4 and out to the count of 8

The addition of the colour to the breathing adds to feelings of calm and takes the focus off the body

Each time you begin counting again, match the count to their breathing

Using the words *'more in control of your relaxation'* ***gives the patient a sense of being in control***

This can be taught in or out of trance as a coping mechanism to control anxious feelings

Breathing through the nose gives additional control and helps to avoid hyperventilation

breathing out the tension ... as I stay silent for a while ... that's it ... ready ... In 2, 3 ... Out 2, 3, 4, 5, 6 ... In 2, 3 ... Out 2, 3, 4, 5, 6 ... breathing in the colour of calm ... breathing out the colour of tension ... In 2, 3 ... Out 2, 3, 4, 5, 6 ... breathe away any tension in your mind ... that's right.

Stay silent for about a minute as you allow the client to continue the rhythm and after a while restart the counting in time with their breathing

Excellent job ... I want you to know that the more you practise this at home ... the more you strengthen the power of this ratio breathing which gives you calm and control in any situation ... any time ... any place ... with anybody you're with ... or just calmly on your own ... calm and control. That's right.

It is useful to set this as a homework activity to practise on a daily basis to reinforce using ratio breathing as a calming coping mechanism

Hand levitation

This also appears in *Calm and confidence for examinations.*

Now you might have heard that the only way to *experience hypnosis* was through the state of relaxation … and of course that is one way you can do it … but you may also be interested to know that you can *go into the hypnotic state through gentle curiosity* … and I know you can *be curious about many different things* … and everybody can be curious to know how the state of mind affects the body and how the body affects the state of mind … and how *some simple changes can be so effective* … and I wonder if you would you be sufficiently curious … and willing … to *experience a change in the state of your hand and fingers* right now? [Pause] Good … so I invite you to rest your fingertips very, very lightly on your knees … that's right … just like this … your fingertips barely touching … and *focus your attention* on just one of those hands … really focus … that's right … keep your gaze on that hand … just focusing … listening …wondering … becoming more and more curious whether it will be what you see … or what you hear … or what you feel … that will enable you to *achieve that wonderful trance state* where *your confidence in yourself increases* … I'd like you to *become very aware of the changes you observe in the hand* … can you notice how … as you look at the hand … you may *find changes beginning to happen?* … It may seem to you that *the hand is becoming fuzzy and blurred* … yes, fuzzy and blurred … or curiously … it may be that the opposite happens … *you may notice a very defined outline around the hand* … becoming more and more defined … interesting I'd like you to … yes, very interesting … *notice these things* and allow yourself to *experience them fully* … in whatever way they occur … for it may be that you *first experience the visual changes* … or it may be that first of all … as you turn your attention now to the weight of the hand … *(or is it lightness?)* … there is an experience of that *hand feeling lighter*

Embedded commands begin immediately in a deceptively conversational way using the inflection of the voice

Generalisation 'everybody can be curious'

'the body affects the state of mind' **seeds the idea that the experience of change (hand levitation) that they are about to experience will affect their state of mind**

Demonstrate how to have the fingertips barely touching the knees

Ratify any response you notice by commenting 'yes that's it' 'that's right' 'interesting' 'Mmm'

'*the* hand' and '*that* hand' **encourages dissociation and a deeper trance state** *and lighter* ... the more you *focus your attention on the sensations in the hand, the more apparent those changes seem to be* ... in fact ... can you *notice the slight tingling in the fingertips?* ... And you can be curious as you notice any little movement ... any little lifting urge ... becoming aware of that *lifting urge* in perhaps one finger ... or is it in more than one finger? ... Or is it *the thumb first* that is wanting to lift higher and higher? ... Or is it *all the fingers* ... as the lightness spreads back into the knuckles? ... A light buoyant feeling now beginning in the palm ... and is the whole hand now feeling lighter as the urge to *lift higher and higher is becoming irresistible* ... as if the hand *has a confident mind* of its own ... as if it can decide all by itself that it *will* lift higher *and higher* as if it's floating ... as indeed it *can* float ... *all on its own ... higher and higher ... all on its own at the unconscious level.* And as you continue to observe the hand floating and lifting all on its own ... aware of the experience of the change in perception of your hand ... you may also become aware of the positive change in your own inner confidence as you also now begin to notice the feeling of heaviness in your eyelids ... how, as the hand gets lighter and lighter ... you can feel that heaviness developing in your eyelids ... heavier and heavier ... as the urge for them to *close* becomes more insistent now ... that's right ... allowing that *wonderful sense of relief to spread over you* as the *eyelids close now* and you *develop that deeper sense of calm hypnotic relaxation.*

There are several phrases in this section which encourage dissociation and depth of the trance state, e.g. *'the thumb' 'all the fingers'* **'the hand** *has a confident mind* **of its own'** 'can decide all by itself'

The very act of hand levitation has an extraordinarily convincing effect

Links a change in the perception of the hand to a change in perception of more positive confidence

Reorientation Procedures

Generally it is useful if a reorientation mirrors an induction: formal inductions with formal reorientations, and informal inductions with informal reorientations.

Use a shift in voice tone to encourage alert reorientation, usually increasing pace of delivery, brightness, and positivity. However, always be sensitive to your client and the type of work you have done together. An abundance of positivity and cheerfulness will not be well accepted from someone dealing with depression or bereavement.

Delivery of suggestions or counting is best done on the in breath, the opposite of how it is carried out in inductions.

Remember to remove suggestions which were made purely for the period of the trance, for example heaviness, lightness, feelings of floating, parts floating out.

In certain cases it would be very useful for clients to feel lighter and brighter so you can suggest that only any *inappropriate* lightness would be removed.

Generally, where you have used parts work, negotiations between parts for change of role or intention for example, suggestions for reintegration of all parts working together for the overall good of the person should be remembered. However, my view is that certain parts may be left in a safe place outside (certainly for a period of time) with the proviso that they may be reaccessed at a time and place of the person's choosing. In the case of pain, for example, a part experiencing the pain may be dissociated as long as it is medically safe to do so. It would then not be sensible to reintegrate this part totally unless it has a change of role, or a suggestion that it can dissociate and reassociate as required.

Suggestions for amnesia or distraction may also be included to inhibit conscious analysis of what has taken place in the trance state.

Reorientation plus conversational reintegration

And I'm wondering ... which aspects of everything that has happened today will be the most pleasing to you ... the most satisfying ... and even the most surprising over the *days and weeks ahead* ... *as perhaps you are wondering too?* And this sense of curiosity will increase over the next few days and weeks as you find *you are noticing the many positive changes in your everyday life* ... and now it is time for you to reorient to the room ... aware of how you *feel so rested and refreshed* ... and *coming back with a deep sense of being at one with yourself* ... *all parts of you working together for your greater good* ... a wonderful sense of satisfaction that *you have finally achieved something* you have been wanting to do for a very long time ... and as you reorient now ... notice the energy coming back into your toes as they want to wriggle about ... yes ... and your fingers too ... that's right ... and feeling that you want to have a good stretch ... that energy spreading all over you now ... wide awake ... very alert ... fully in the moment ... invigorated ... looking forward to the day ahead ... Welcome back!

This leads them to begin 'wondering'

Embedded command to notice the forthcoming changes

Conversational reintegration

Focuses on satisfaction and presupposes that something positive has been achieved

Suggestions for becoming re-energised

Orienting the client to the future

302

Energising

And in a few moments, it will be time for you to begin that process of reorienting to your surroundings and … just before you do … take a few moments to reflect on the changes begun … or perhaps even already completed in you … here today … either … or both … consciously or unconsciously … and it's good to know that these changes will have a positive effect on your life over forthcoming days and weeks and months … and please congratulate yourself for what you have achieved. [Pause]

One of these achievements is the effect of a deep inner relaxation which leaves you feeling refreshed and renewed … not only physically but emotionally and mentally too … you can experience an energy that will inspire you over the coming days/weeks/months ... a little like a wellspring inside with all the resources you need … overflowing into every part of you … every part of you *sensing this energy* in its own special way … knowing there are things to think about … things to *feel enthusiastic about … things to set in motion* … I'm wondering how you will first *become aware of this physical energy in you* … this excitement in you … *even now noticing an urge for your fingers and toes to wriggle about* … perhaps *a desire to stretch … your eyelids fluttering and becoming excited to open* … becoming wider and wider awake and alert … all parts of you refreshed, re-energised and revitalised … almost as though you have had the most amazing sleep … all parts working in harmony together as you *open your eyes now* ... welcome back ... it's going to be such a wonderful day. You are going to *ensure it's a wonderful day*!

Introduces the idea of reorientation and gives a time for them to reinforce changes already initiated

Use enthusiasm and energy in your own voice and speed up delivery

Reframe energy as excitement

Conversational reintegration

Unconscious continuation

You have started a process here today which will *continue at many levels* ... there will undoubtedly be conscious decisions that are made and, underlying these, will be unconscious processes which occur without your necessarily being aware of them ... rather like what happens when you try and try consciously to remember the name of someone but it just won't come to mind ... but later ... seemingly out of nowhere ... you suddenly recall that name because your unconscious mind has been continuing its search while you were involved in something else entirely ... just as *you will find in the forthcoming hours/days/weeks ... ideas/solutions/resolutions/ realisations will occur to you* ... some may be surprising and some seem quite obvious and some may be quite transformational ... but all of these will *satisfy a need in you at some level and will be life enhancing* ... so, as you *begin to reorient to the room now* ... I'm wondering how you will *become aware of this energy in you* ... not only in your body but also in your inner self/in your spirit/in your soul ... *at first already noticing an urge for your fingers and toes to wriggle about* ... perhaps *a desire to stretch* ... *your eyelids becoming excited to open* ... and you ... *feeling a great sense of curiosity as to how soon and exactly what interesting results of unconscious processes you will be noticing that will affect you so positively in a whole variety of ways* ... are you also wondering how this difference in you will be noticed by those people around you? ... And so now reorienting completely with a sense of inner harmony and positivity ... all parts of you working together for your greater good ... becoming wider and wider awake and alert ... refreshed, re-energised and revitalised as you *open your eyes now* ... welcome back.

Gives an everyday example of unconscious processes at work

Presupposition that this energy exists

Other people observing someone's new behaviour is thought to act as strong reinforcement of that behaviour

Post-pain relief scripts

This ending also occurs in the script *Leave the pain beside you.*

So now it's time for you to *reorient to the room* …
every part of you understanding its very own special
role for you … keeping you just as comfortable as
can be … isn't it good to *know that your unconscious mind and your body can do this together …
knowing exactly when and which parts to let rest or
even sleep for a while* … allowing your body's own
innate forces to produce their natural calming and
comforting endorphins while doing their wonderful healing work … gently returning to conscious
awareness of *how much more rested you feel …
how much more comfortable you feel … how much
you have calmed and taken control of your thoughts*
… gently … comfortably coming back now … with
*that sense of optimism … in a rather unusual way
… being experienced in your body as well as in your
mind* … a strong sense of being *focused on positive
ideas and experiences … a feeling of being uplifted
and supported* wherever you are … whenever you're
there … whomever you're with or simply when
you're comfortably and easily enjoying your own
company … that's it … refreshed and well rested …
welcome back.

Some parts can be rested
or allowed to sleep, e.g.
the parts which experience
chronic pain or parts which
have been temporarily
dissociated through
negotiation

Presuppositions of greater
well-being and optimism

305

Positive focus, ego strengthening and conversational reorientation

So the really important thing to be fully aware of at this moment is that you have started an amazing process here today (for which congratulations) which will continue over the forthcoming days, weeks and months ... and you will *speed up and strengthen that process* the more often you *use your mind consciously to direct your positive future*. The more you *focus on exactly what you want to happen, getting a mental picture with lots of vibrant detail and talking yourself confidently through the situation* ... the more you will be able to trust your inner mind to *carry out your wishes* and help you *create your own brighter future. The more often you practise thinking optimistically with your conscious mind ... the more optimistic you will become deep inside,* and the more you will find you are increasingly able to cope with any situation you face in your everyday life ... cope with anybody ... cope with anything so much more confidently than ever you thought you could ... and just as soon as your conscious mind and your unconscious mind have found the way to work in harmony to *ensure all of this happens* ... just as I know it will ... you will *begin to notice the energy now beginning to spread around your body* ... your fingers perhaps beginning to notice it first ... then your hands and arms wanting to stretch ... and as your body is feeling this, it reflects the energy present and growing in your mind to get on with improving your life in so many ways ... and your eyelids beginning to flutter as they are wanting to open as you reorient to the room, completely alert and aware of the feeling of optimism growing inside that feels really good. Welcome back ... every tiny part of you fully in the present moment in the room with me ... feeling good! And looking very calm/confident/relaxed/energised/refreshed too!

Congratulations validate and reinforce change
'which will continue'

Gives suggestion for ongoing conscious practice of positive thinking

Ego strengthening

Conscious and unconscious co-operation

Suggestions for re-energising body and mind

Suggestions for physical movement will cause it to happen and comments on any perceived movement will encourage more of it to occur. Comment as appropriate

Positive focus with a strong urge to put plans into action

Very appropriate after goal-setting-type scripts and for any coaching situations.

So congratulations on having made some interesting and very useful discoveries (about the way you think/respond/feel about/do things) and I'd like to remind you that your unconscious mind is extraordinarily powerful and will … not only continue the process of honing, refining and finalising the plans that you have started to make today … but it will also help you *carry out all these plans and suggestions once they have been finalised* … and even more than that … it will *continue to motivate you long after this session is over*. Very soon … if not already … you will begin to *become aware of a sense of reorienting to your surroundings* … a sense of energy coming back into your body as well as into your mind … can you already perhaps *notice a sense of wanting to stretch?* … A sense of excitement too as you realise that *you just want to get on with things* … a sense of positive urgency to make things happen … a need to get things done now and not just talk about them … and … as that sense grows … your eyelids are beginning to flutter as they want to open … and you know that as soon as they do *open wide now* … you will have this feeling of being on a mission … there are things you need to do … nothing will stop you … you will do whatever is right … whatever is positive … whatever is forward moving … and in a good way … you will do whatever it takes to make it happen. Great, your eyes are opening and you are certainly *looking* good … tell me how you *feel!*

Presupposition

A reminder that the process will continue contains an implicit suggestion to expect ongoing positive changes

Use your voice to encourage the idea of excitement and positivity

Use the emphasis of your voice to compare how the client *looks* and how they *feel*

Healing

As you reorient to the room you can be aware that every part of you involved in the healing process will *be active and vigilant over the upcoming days/weeks/months* ... they will *continue restoring, renewing, and doing their healing work physically and emotionally throughout the day and night* ... and ... do know that your body's healing forces do a great deal of their healing work while you sleep ... you will *sleep quietly and comfortably through the night* ... getting all the rest you need and in the morning you will *wake refreshed and revitalised* ... each morning there will be a growing sense ... in mind, body and spirit ... of positive anticipation for the day ahead ... and even now ... you are beginning to be aware of this as you reorient to the room ... an eagerness to *enjoy the day in the best way for you* ... feeling a sense of relief/contentment/gratitude/confidence that your body understands how to heal naturally ... all at the unconscious level ... leaving you free to use your conscious mind to *engage in any enjoyable activity you want* ... all parts of your conscious and unconscious working in harmony for your overall well-being ... feeling the energy now coming back into the body ... first in the fingers perhaps ... (or is it the toes?) ... a feeling of wanting to stretch and get on with your day ... a feeling of being refreshed and revitalised in your whole body as you come back to the room with me ... you have this wonderful feeling that things are going to go very well today as you *allow your eyes to open and reorient to your surroundings* ... welcome back ... you do look very refreshed!

Reassuring to know that the processes of healing are ongoing

Let your voice become progressively more lively as you continue

308

Suggestions you may wish to include in any chosen reorientation

Removal of phenomena induced purely for the duration of the trance

And when you reorient to the room … you will find that any inappropriate lightness or heaviness in your body … will be lifted from you and every part throughout your whole body will have comfort, ease, and full extent of movement. If there is lightness, it will be that lightness of spirit that you are experiencing after this liberating/positive/empowering experience here today.

Keep the benefit of insights/learning/changes with a degree of amnesia for how they came about

As you reorient to your surroundings you will keep all these insights/learning/changes in a special place in you where your unconscious will make use of them in the best possible way … and you may or may not remember the detail at the conscious level … the important thing is that you will *remember to notice that you are experiencing the benefits of them* although the exact 'whys and wherefores' may elude you … and you find yourself feeling very comfortable with that.

Distraction

And later … once fully reoriented to surroundings and full alert waking state … some people find that they try to recall that intriguing trance state … they try really hard to explain the thoughts and images and the things that were said … but somehow those things elude them even though they know that they were important and they get that feeling deep within that there's been a change for the better … remarkable even … they say it's like the beginning of springtime … when there's renewal of hope … the urge to move forward … there's light to see more clearly … feel a spring in the step … an enthusiasm for life itself that you can sense when you see the buds on the trees … ideas straining to burst into life … so time for you to begin that reorientation now and experience this new beginning in whichever way is right for you.

References and Useful Resources

I have only referred directly to the work of one author, Michael Yapko in this volume in relation to his work in using hypnosis in the treatment of depression (the section of *Mild to Moderate Depression*).

Time management and procrastination

Some ideas were inspired by Martin Scott in his book mentioned below.

Sport and performance

Some ideas were inspired by John Edgette and Tim Rowan in their book mentioned below. Also talks by Anne Smith at the APHP Conference and by Alma Thomas at the London College of Clinical Hypnosis

The other books are those that have been influential in my own hypnotherapy work and those that I would recommend most highly.

Boyne, Gil. (1989) *Transforming Therapy; a New Approach to Hypnotherapy*. Westwood Publishing Company, Inc. USA

Bryant, Mike and Mabbutt, Peter. (2006) *Hypnotherapy for Dummies*. John Wiley and Sons. UK
[A useful book for the general public and a quick reference for trainee hypnotherapists.]

Edgette, John H. and Rowan, Tim. (2003) *Winning the Mind Game*. Crown House Publishing Ltd. UK and USA

Haven, Ronald A. and Walters, Catherine. (1989) *Hypnotherapy Scripts*. Brunner/Mazel. USA

Hunter, Marlene E. (1994) *Creative Scripts for Hypnotherapy*. Brunner/Mazel. USA

Hunter, Roy (2005) *Hypnosis for Inner Conflict Resolution*. Crown House Publishing Ltd. UK

James, Ursula. (2005) *Clinical Hypnosis Textbook*. Radcliffe Publishing Ltd. UK

Joseph, Avy. (2009) *Cognitive Behavioural Therapy; your Route out of Perfectionism, Self Sabotage and Other Everyday Habits.* Capstone Publishing Ltd. UK

Overdurf, John and Silverthorne, Julie. (1994) *Training Trances.* Metamorphous Press. USA

Scott, Martin. (1998) *More Time, Less Stress.* Century Ltd. UK

Watts, Terence. (2005) *Hypnosis: Advanced Techniques of Hypnotherapy and Hypnoanalysis.* Network 3000 Publishing. USA

Yapko, Michael D. (1992) *Hypnosis and the Treatment of Depressions.* Brunner/Mazel. USA

Yapko, Michael D. (2001) *Treating Depression with Hypnosis Integrating Cognitive-Behavioural and Strategic Approaches.* Brunner-Routledge. USA

I am grateful to Jeffrey Zeig for inspiring me with the idea of 'cushions of calm' which he used in one of his hypnosis workshops. I have subsequently used cushions of all kinds of inner resources in my therapy work.

Jeffrey K. Zeig. The Milton Erickson Foundation. www.Jeffzeig.com

www.firstwayforward.com Information on one day seminars by the author, Lynda Hudson plus a wide selection of hypnotherapy CDs and digital downloads